Contents

Why we wrote THE NO CRAVE DIET

As a naturopathic doctor (Penny) and an orthopaedic surgeon (Steve), we represent opposite ends of the medical spectrum. As such, we're are often asked not only how we find common ground to write together, but also how we stay married (ten years this summer!). The answer is simple: we believe in using a range of treatments, incorporating natural and traditional therapy, to both treat and prevent illness. We respect each other's profession and practise in a way that provides the best management of our patients.

Over the past ten years we have seen research on weight gain and energy metabolism emerge from small studies in isolated laboratories into mainstream medical investigation. Fuelled by funding from governments anxious to stem the growing impact of weight-related illness on their economies, and pharmaceutical companies who visualize the Holy Grail of 'fat-busting' medicine, scientists throughout the world have made tremendous progress towards answering the many questions that surround weight gain and dieting. We have followed this research with interest and, by combining it with the naturopathic principles used in our day-to-day practice, have formulated a plan that our patients swear by. Many of them have tried numerous diets before with limited success or they have regained the lost weight as soon as they strayed.

All books require inspiration and this is no exception. As with all of our books, we write to bring our message to a far wider audience than we could ever reach through our practices.

It's incredibly rewarding to watch people liberate themselves from the tortuous cycle of cravings and failed diets; to be able to regain control of what they eat and achieve and maintain their ideal weight. Even more fulfilling is the knowledge that they will be happier and much healthier as a result – even live longer because of it.

Penny says: My initial idea for THE NO CRAVE DIET came from one of my patients. She had seen me in my office for weight loss and had been using my notes and hand-outs for a number of months. Already well into Phase-2 of my plan, and down about 3 stones (19kg), she asked why I hadn't put all my information into a book. It seemed like the perfect next step. I had been using the diet with my patients with great success for a few years and I knew it was based on sound research. In addition, the basic science behind the diet, including the brain's control of hunger and craving, were beginning to make their way into magazines and newspapers. With THE NO CRAVE DIET, once we explain how food cravings and the tendency to gain weight are related, we can start you on a diet, supplement and lifestyle plan that reverses the unhealthy imbalance within your body. The book incorporates the basic principles of our No-Crave Diet, updated with current medical research to improve its effectiveness, reduce food cravings and promote fat burning. In addition, we use a number of safe, readily available, natural supplements to support you and further decrease cravings. Simple lifestyle changes address issues such as stress, which plays a large role in both food cravings and weight gain.

Most of our patients notice a significant reduction in their food cravings within 48 hours and an average weight loss of 2 pounds per week.

Steve says: **Of course, the obvious question is why an orthopaedic surgeon is writing a diet book. There are two main reasons. The first is my interest in improving health, a vision I share with Penny and the basis behind our books. The second is that it offers significant benefits to my patients. Even as a surgeon, surgery remains the last option for many orthopaedic problems, particularly arthritis. Other non-surgical treatments should always be tried first and in cases where it is appropriate, weight loss is exceedingly effective at reducing pain, particularly from the hips and knees. Even in individuals awaiting surgery, weight loss improves the outcome and reduces complications.**

THE NO CRAVE DIET represents the culmination of five years of research and clinical practice and allows the reader to follow a diet we have used successfully with our patients. We believe in simple communication and have made it as easy to understand and follow as it would be for individuals we were looking after personally.

We wish you success and good health.

PART I
Introduction

What are food cravings?

Food cravings are the reason we cheat on our diet. They are responsible for everything from nibbling on a tasty snack to succumbing to the chocolate cheesecake at the end of an otherwise perfectly healthy meal. Food cravings are all about reward, making you feel good in the short term but inevitably bad in the long run.

Diets are, in general, not renowned for making you feel particularly buoyant, so not surprisingly you crave a treat once in a while. The harder you diet, the stronger the cravings. You know you don't really need that snack but the little voice in your head is telling you just one can't hurt. You concoct excuses to justify it and eventually you give in: the start of a slippery slope, down which your diet slides away.

But food cravings and that voice in your head have nothing to do with you needing more calories. They are just messages from your brain, tricking you into providing it with a reward. Your brain wants to feel good – and who can blame it! Whenever the going gets a little tough – a stressful event, an emotional crisis or even a new diet – it remembers those tasty treats and conditions you to hunt them out.

But by understanding these cravings and learning to recognise their causes you can counteract them. By satisfying the brain in other ways you can actually turn off its little voice and begin to diet without suffering.

How food cravings disrupt your diet

It's estimated that 80 per cent of diets fail because people give in to food cravings. Whatever weight-loss plan you follow the desire to snack invariably overwhelms even the most ardent and determined dieter. It starts with just the one chip and before long the diet you were on is a distant memory and any weight lost is regained. That little voice tempting you to cheat is a powerful force, not only giving you food cravings but finding excuses and toying with your emotions, making you feel tired, even unwell, grouchy or depressed, wearing you down until you find yourself snacking, grazing or making a midnight trip to the fridge!

But what if you could silence that voice, banish those cravings and unpleasant feelings of hunger? Suddenly your diet would become painless. You would no longer dread each day, hoping one less pound on the scales will justify the suffering. Instead, because you would no longer be constantly tempted to cheat by having a snack, the pounds would come off and you could stick to your diet until you decided to stop.

And what if you discovered that the same factors causing you to experience these food cravings were also inhibiting your ability to burn fat? Well, it's true: by addressing one problem you automatically fix the other – double whammy!

Why controlling food cravings is the new direction in weight loss

THE **NO CRAVE** DIET, a mixture of dietary and lifestyle changes, will enable you to lose weight without all the unpleasant side effects normally associated with dieting.

Previous diet plans have relied solely on calories or food types, but the No-Crave plan is based on research into how the brain controls our hunger, research that has shown us which biological processes make it so difficult to resist cheating, so difficult to make rational food choices and stay faithful to a weight-loss programme. No diet can be effective if you cannot stick to it.

But by countering the biological processes that make us crave the wrong foods, the No-Crave plan will actually make it easy for you to stick to your diet. You will no longer be tempted to snack or cheat simply because you will no longer be overwhelmed by the urge.

The plan incorporates all the things that affect our ability to lose weight – not only the nutritional ones but also biological and psychological reasons that previous diet plans haven't taken into account. My patients come to my clinic in desperation, because they can't stick to a diet, whichever one they try; no matter how effective it may be, in practice it doesn't work because they can't remain faithful to the plan. But once on the No-Crave plan 90 per cent of my patients notice a significant reduction in their food cravings within 48 hours, and they lose on average two pounds per week. This simple plan can be used as a diet in its own right or as an aid to any existing diet. And apart from banishing your cravings there are many other benefits. By altering the processes that cause your cravings you will automatically be switching your metabolism to fat-burning rather than fat-storing mode. And there are multiple health benefits, as I will explain.

Tackling food cravings is the key to losing weight:

They are the most likely cause of failure with any diet because they make you cheat and snack

• •

Cravings give you a taste for unhealthy foods, instead of nutritious ones

• •

Cravings lead to snacking, and snacking reduces the amount of fat your body can burn between meals

• •

Giving in to food cravings traps you in a vicious cycle, leading to more cravings

• •

Intense cravings cause stress and unhealthy emotions such as depression and guilt

What happens when we experience food cravings?

A craving begins with a deep-seated ache somewhere just below your ribcage and the inability to rid yourself of intrusive thoughts about a certain type of food. These feelings can be so intense, some people say they can actually smell or taste the food they crave. Such a craving rapidly takes over your day as you either try to battle it out or search for the appropriate snack to satisfy it. There is no logic to a craving. You may have eaten only half an hour ago, it may not even be a food you typically eat, but once it hits it seems to be the only thing you will ever want to eat again.

Many things cause cravings but calorie-restriction diets typically increase cravings, which is why they are so hard to follow. And the stress brought on by cravings not only makes your diet hard work, but also actually induces further cravings – stress-induced cravings. To make matters even worse, the foods we crave for are unhealthy ones (let's face it, it's rare to crave a celery stick mid-afternoon), the very foods that stimulate our brains to want more of these food types – food-induced cravings.

This is how food cravings trap us within a vicious cycle of craving and snacking, and because eating too regularly prevents the body from switching on its fat-burning system, the fat stays where it is. Cravings are the ultimate in dietary sabotage!

So what happens when we get a food craving? While it may seem that the feelings are centred in our stomach the actual process behind the craving starts in our brain. And like any good story there is good and evil, in this case hunger and satiety, with satiety being the comfortable, non-hungry state you experience at the end of a meal. The balance between the two is delicate and when the pendulum swings towards hunger, the cravings take over and your whole body is forced to succumb to food-finding behaviour. It is a primitive force, quite ruthless once unleashed, with plenty of tricks and turns to ensure battling it is an uphill task.

Why you feel hungry

Our appetite and ability to lose weight hangs in the balance, the outcome dependent on who wins the battle for control over whether we feel hungry or full.

What is hunger?

Hunger is an emptiness in the stomach, an increase in rumblings, a little light-headedness. We think about food, we become more agitated, highly attuned to sights or smells, and we start to plan our next meal or snack.

What is satiety?

Satiety – the sensation of feeling 'full' – is a little less familiar. Some may only consider it that uncomfortable feeling at the end of an overly large supper requiring the belt to be let out a notch. Other sensations include calmness or even sleepiness, loss of interest in food or even distaste.

These feelings are being controlled not by your stomach or your fat cells but by your brain!

Hunger and the brain

Our brain contains a hunger centre that makes us feel hungry and a satiety centre that makes us feel full. The hunger centre tells us to find and eat food. Remember how you feel at your most famished, thinking of food, imagining your next meal, barely able to concentrate on anything else. This is your hunger centre firing on all cylinders.

EMPTY

Your hunger centre

- Makes you feel hungry
- Encourages you to look for food
- Encourages your body to store energy
- Increases fat storing
- Reduces fat burning
- Slows you down by limiting your energy supply
- Turns down the body's mechanism of creating heat by burning fat

Hunger switched on
Search for food
Eat
Save energy
Store fat

HUNGER CENTRE

The satiety centre, on the other hand, switches off the desire to eat, reduces your desire to snack and actually promotes fat burning.

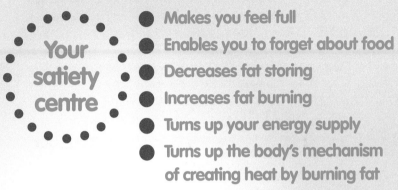

Your satiety centre

- Makes you feel full
- Enables you to forget about food
- Decreases fat storing
- Increases fat burning
- Turns up your energy supply
- Turns up the body's mechanism of creating heat by burning fat

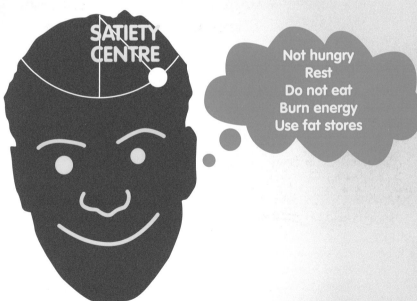

SATIETY CENTRE

Not hungry
Rest
Do not eat
Burn energy
Use fat stores

There is a tug-of-war in the brain between our hunger centre and our satiety centre. Certain factors swing the pendulum either towards hunger, eating and fat storage or towards satiety and fat burning.

What makes us feel hungry or full?

Brain research has shown that the overwhelming drive within the brain is to seek out food and eat it. Hunger is our natural state: the hunger centre remains active and the brain hungry until sufficient satiety messages are received from our body. These satiety messages inform the brain everything is fine out here, we have enough energy, we can relax – for a while. The satiety centre becomes active enough to counteract the hunger centre and temporarily reduce our desire to eat. This mechanism is essentially a residual primitive response, designed for the foraging caveman, preventing complacency about hunting down the next meal. Sadly for us, the system is not quite so useful in an environment where food is available 24–7 in a form where the only hunting required is for a parking spot!

The direction of the pendulum is determined by a number of things – not only dietary changes but also emotional, physical and metabolic changes. By learning what makes the pendulum swing, we can learn how to influence its direction in favour of satiety so that we switch off our hunger for longer periods.

Hardwired to be hungry – blood sugar

Simply being on a diet is enough to induce food cravings. Your brain is already hardwired to be hungry, a throwback to our primitive days when food was scarce. Going on a diet, particularly one that involves fasting or calorie deprivation, immediately enhances that drive, causing the hunger centre of the brain to go into overdrive. The same is true for low blood sugar or hypoglycaemia, another side effect of a poorly designed diet.

The hunger centre responds quickly to falling blood sugar by stimulating our desire to seek out food, particularly sweet snacks that rapidly return our blood sugar to normal. Unfortunately as soon as we eat the sugary treat our body releases large amounts of insulin, which sweeps the sugar out of our bloodstream and stores it as fat. Our blood sugar drops again and the food cravings return. By stabilising blood sugar, THE NO CRAVE DIET eliminates one of the key causes of food cravings.

Reward

We often snack as a reward, not necessarily as a prize for having achieved some incredible feat, but because we all need a treat once in a while. It makes us feel good because our brain has an in-built circuit that responds positively to reward. When this reward circuit is balanced we experience a sense of satisfied calm and pleasure; when it is not balanced it starts controlling our behaviour, making us do what is necessary to restore its balance.

Most of us have taught our reward centre that the quickest way to restore balance and feel happy once more is to satisfy a food craving, therefore it instructs us to seek out a snack. The drive can be remarkably strong; some of the chemicals involved in this reward process are similar to morphine, so it is not surprising that most of us eventually succumb.

THE NO CRAVE DIET enables you to remove your dependence on food as a treat and to retrain your behaviour so that you focus less on reward.

Certain foods generate craving

Some of the foods we eat actually keep our hunger switched on. Snacks high in sugar or fat make the hunger centre more active and override our normal control mechanisms. By swinging the balance in favour of hunger rather than satiety we are driven to eat bigger portions and to eat for longer periods, so we eat more than we need to, and gain weight.

Another food that keeps your hunger switched on is an ingredient used to sweeten many fast foods, processed foods or quickly prepared meals. It is called high-fructose corn syrup. It is not recognised by the satiety centre and therefore does not switch off your hunger. So despite the large number of calories consumed with these meals you still feel hungry.

THE NO CRAVE DIET teaches you which foods and ingredients increase cravings, and which ones keep you feeling full.

Stress makes you hungry

Stress increases hunger and snacking in several ways. Although the stress response is supposed to protect us from danger, it is designed for the occasional escape from a marauding animal, not the continuous assault of finances, work, commuting, family and multitasking. Each time an acute stress response is over, our brain and metabolism shift into recovery mode, to replace all that energy we expended while sprinting to safety. We feel hungry, seek food and eat. Sadly, however stressful our commute to work, sitting in the car for an hour hardly burns excess calories. So the extra food we are inclined to eat, once this stress of the commute is over, heads straight to our fat stores.

Another way in which stress leads to cravings is by making you unhappy. When the stress response is being activated continuously, as with chronic stress, the stress hormone, cortisol, reduces our happy hormone, serotonin, which leads us to desire those fatty sugary foods that rapidly make us feel good again.

Furthermore, the stress hormone cortisol raises our blood sugar in much the same way a biscuit would. And as with a biscuit, the subsequent drop in blood sugar, caused by insulin release, leads to food craving. Cortisol also increases addictive behaviour, enhancing our tendency to seek out more and more rewarding snacks.

These are just some of the ways in which stress increases our cravings. And research has shown us how this occurs in animals too. Rats exposed to chronic stress calm themselves by selecting comfort foods high in sugar and fat.

THE NO CRAVE DIET reduces and controls the stress response so you feel calmer on your diet and are able to face the day's endeavours without risking a stress-induced snack.

Emotions and comfort eating

Emotional upheaval increases hunger. Feeling low or depressed is one of the commonest triggers for food cravings. Even a happy event often causes a reactive low afterwards, and we eat to try and regain the high. The main culprit here is our happy hormone, serotonin. Low levels are linked with depression. When our serotonin is low we feel sluggish, apathetic, sad and weepy. But serotonin is released when we eat chocolate, sweet foods or the type of carbohydrates that break down quickly into sugar, so when we eat these foods it makes us feel relaxed and elated. This is why we crave sweets and starches when we are depressed, and also why women crave these foods when their serotonin levels dip just before a period.

THE NO CRAVE DIET reduces the impact of these emotion-induced cravings while maximising levels of our happy hormone.

Let's talk turkey

Serotonin is made from the amino acid tryptophan and certain foods, such as turkey, are tryptophan-rich. Hence the need for a post-Christmas-lunch snooze. Unfortunately, a slice of turkey is not nearly as accessible as a chocolate bar when we need that serotonin!

Midnight munchies and the anti-hunger hormone

The anti-hunger hormone leptin switches off our hunger. It normally gets released overnight to enable us to sleep; otherwise our hunger would wake us up.

But we can develop resistance to this anti-hunger hormone, particularly when we are overweight, and when we develop this resistance it not only makes us feel hungry despite having plenty of reserves in our fat stores, but also prevents our hunger being switched off at night, so we find ourselves making a surreptitious midnight or early-morning trip to the fridge in search of a snack to satisfy the craving that is keeping us awake.

THE NO CRAVE DIET reverses the abnormal resistance to leptin, allowing it to effectively shut off your hunger centre.

The hunger messenger and why a big lunch doesn't make you less hungry later

Levels of the hunger messenger ghrelin are raised by having an empty stomach, inducing extreme feelings of hunger and food-seeking behaviour. These strong food cravings are almost impossible to ignore. Unfortunately eating a large lunch in order to make you less hungry at dinner doesn't work, because ghrelin levels are not influenced by the size of your last meal and may even be increased by a substantial feasting. And being overweight can impair your body's ability to switch off this hunger hormone, even when your stomach is full.

THE NO CRAVE DIET controls ghrelin by providing adequate meal size and slower stomach emptying so you feel less hungry between meals. Correct food choices and meal timing reduces the hunger-inducing effect of ghrelin.

Snacking increases snacking

Finally, as if there is not enough stacked against us, snacking actually causes more snacking. Research shows that giving in to our cravings actually exacerbates them. Not convinced? Try opening a bag of crisps and eating just one.

THE NO CRAVE DIET will break this vicious cycle of snacking.

Counter the cravings to lose weight

So you can see why even the most determined dieter becomes overwhelmed by the desire for their favourite tasty foods or snacks, and why food cravings are the reason most diets fail. It is hard to ignore these powerful brain messengers – that little voice telling you that one biscuit can't hurt. But with THE NO CRAVE DIET you can counter this voice by swinging the pendulum more towards your brain's satiety centre and less towards your brain's hunger centre. THE NO CRAVE DIET will show you how to beat your cravings so you can lose weight.

The top ⑩ reasons we get food cravings

- When we reduce the number of calories we eat, we automatically increase our hunger by increasing activity in the hunger centre
- Low blood sugar from poor food choices promotes hunger and snacking
- We like to reward ourselves with snacks as it makes us feel good, the effect of the brain's in-built incentive programme
- Sugary or fatty foods actually promote snacking and the desire for more foods of this type
- Ongoing daily stress increases hunger and the seeking out of comfort foods
- Emotional upheaval, feeling low or depressed leads us to seek out snacks that will increase our brain's happy hormone, serotonin
- The hormonal changes associated with PMS (premenstrual syndrome) cause major food cravings
- Resistance to the fat hormone leptin leads to snacking and the midnight munchies
- Large meals or being overweight can increase levels of the hunger hormone ghrelin, making us feel more hungry
- Snacking itself leads to more snacking – the reason it is so hard to have just one crisp or one biscuit

PART II
The No-Crave Diet Plan

Following **THE NO CRAVE DIET** plan enables you to switch off your cravings and shows you how to return to eating a varied and tasty diet without getting caught in a vicious cycle of recurrent cravings and regaining the weight you lost. Not only does this make the diet easier to stick to, it makes it more successful, by increasing your fat-burning potential and rebalancing your metabolism so the food you eat is used as fuel rather than stored as fat. This sounds as if it is asking a lot of a diet, but it is in fact rather straightforward, as well as being simple and painless to institute. And your health will not suffer. On the contrary, your health will actually improve.

Although the No-Crave plan offers many ways to combat cravings, such as supplements and simple lifestyle exercises, the diet part of the plan itself also reduces the desire to snack.

The first phase is a weight-loss plan that also weans you off snacking, quells food cravings and rebalances your metabolism. This first phase lasts from six to eight weeks, depending on your body size. The second phase is the maintenance phase, in which your dietary choices expand; restricted items are reintroduced, allowing you the freedom to enjoy many different types of food without regaining the weight you lost in Phase 1.

Benefits of THE NO CRAVE DIET

- Minimise your food cravings
- Lose weight safely and healthily
- Rebalance your metabolism to:
  - Use your food as fuel rather than store it as fat
  - Increase your fat-burning potential
- Improve your health
- Reduce your risk of disease

Basic principles of No-Crave eating

There are two key elements to No-Crave eating: changing what you eat and changing when you eat.

Changing what you eat
Changing what you eat reduces food cravings by:

- Stabilising your blood sugar
- Rebalancing your metabolism, which reduces snacking
- Keeping you feeling fuller for longer
- Improving your access to your body's stores
- Reducing your desire for foods that increase cravings
- Avoiding foods that promote cravings
- Reducing your sugar and fat intake, leading to less snacking

Changing when you eat
Changing when you eat reduces food cravings by:

- Stabilising your blood sugar
- Optimising the action of insulin
- Maximising the energy function of your liver
- Allowing leptin to turn off your hunger

The key to successful weight loss without cravings is 'NO SNACKING' and once you rid yourself of food cravings this will be easy. THE **NO CRAVE DIET** consists of three meals per day. The concept of eating every few hours ignores some of the basic science behind metabolism and weight loss. We are simply not designed to have meals five or six times a day. Our metabolism and biochemistry is essentially unchanged from our caveman days, a time when even two meals per day would have been a luxury. Prehistoric man was certainly not lounging about in his cave, one hand tucked into the waistband of his loin cloth, the other reaching into a bowl of pterodactyl wings every couple of hours. Meals were scarce, and subsequently we remain most efficient with a maximum of three meals a day. These comprise a good breakfast, five or six hours until lunch, another five or six before dinner and then eleven or twelve until our next breakfast.

Meal timing on the No-Crave Diet

BREAKFAST

LUNCH

DINNER

Midnight 1am 2am 3am 4am 5am 6am 7am 8am 9am 10am 11am Noon 1pm 2pm 3pm 4pm 5pm 6pm 7pm 8pm 9pm 10pm 11pm Midnight

The graph shows a range of possible meal times, but keep to your No-Crave schedule. If you eat breakfast at 8 a.m. you cannot start lunch at 11 a.m. – you must wait until 12.30 or 1 p.m.

Depending on your daily schedule, meal times may be different from those suggested above. However, there must be five to six hours between breakfast and lunch, another five to six hours between lunch and dinner and eleven to twelve hours between dinner and breakfast.

The No-Crave eating plan will ease you into this no-snacking routine by eliminating mid-morning and mid-afternoon hunger pangs, and by changing when you eat to three meals a day with no snacks you will improve your ability to burn fat stores and lose weight, because fat-burning typically begins three hours after a meal. It will also eliminate late-night munchies. It is important not to succumb to midnight munchies if you are looking to lose weight, because night-time is a prime time for fat burning.

The two phases of THE **NO CRAVE** DIET

Phase 1 – weight loss

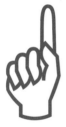

- Corrects metabolic imbalance
- Controls cravings
- Allows healthy weight loss

Phase 2 – healthy maintenance

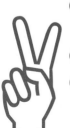

- Maintains your weight while reintro-ducing a full range of food types
- Improves your energy and health
- Controls cravings

THE NO CRAVE DIET is safe and healthy

It is important to understand that THE NO CRAVE DIET is not a low-carbohydrate diet, nor is it a high-protein diet. It is a balanced carbohydrate-to-protein diet with protein levels catered towards each individual.

Most people think of carbohydrates as only including grains, starches and sweet foods such as breads, pastas, rice, bananas and chocolate. However, the most important carbohydrates of all are the vegetables and salads. Yes, that is correct: broccoli is actually a carbohydrate that breaks down into sugar. The difference is that these good carbohydrates (the vegetables and salads) only break down into sugar very slowly. They also provide an important source of many vitamins, minerals and fibre not found in other carbohydrates. Vegetables and salads are permitted in unlimited quantity on the THE NO CRAVE DIET. Also, in limited quantities, most fruits, dressings, condiments and carbohydrates are allowed. So you see, you are actually eating an essentially unlimited-carbohydrate diet.

As far as protein goes, although you may be eating more protein than you were before on this diet, you are only consuming one gram of protein per kilogram (or 2.2lb) of body weight (see chart on page 32). A high-protein diet, such as the Atkins Diet, enforces twice this amount of protein.

The balance of protein to good carbohydrates is what matters and because this weight-loss programme is nutritionally balanced, it is safe for anyone: children, adolescents, the elderly and even those with kidney disease. There is no ketosis, no starvation, no extremes at all. THE NO CRAVE DIET is the safest and most effective permanent weight-loss and health plan to date. You will be eating a more nutritious meal plan than ever before. All your high-calorie low-nutrient carbohydrates such as chips and potatoes are temporarily replaced with nutrient-dense salads, vegetables and fruits.

And any food avoided during Phase 1 can be added back in when you have lost your weight, without fear of regaining weight, and without stimulating further cravings that force you to overindulge. So it is not the No-Eat-Forever Diet, nor is it the No-Fun Diet, it is simply the diet that allows you to eat unlimited carbohydrates along with your favourite proteins, all the while losing weight and shutting off food cravings.

Chapter 1: Phase 1

This phase involves a limited period of time, for two reasons. Firstly, it usually takes six to eight weeks to retrain the body's metabolism. During these weeks, each time you eat protein your body receives a message that your blood-sugar levels are low so it does not need to secrete too much insulin. Once the body has practised and consolidated this message for a period of time it learns to always respond to protein in this way, so you can introduce more carbohydrates with your protein but your insulin will still remain low. Protein will always act as a cue to keep your insulin release small, which will maintain weight loss.

The second reason for keeping Phase 1 down to eight weeks is that after this time you will be likely to have lost enough weight to enjoy a wide variety of healthy foods without fear of regaining it.

Thirdly, although there is essentially no limit to the length of time you can stay in Phase 1, you will probably stop losing weight once your excess fat has been eradicated, and on average this takes around eight weeks. But if after eight weeks you have more weight to lose you can continue with Phase 1 for as long as it takes, without adversely affecting your health.

The good news is that after the first six to eight weeks, cheating or straying temporarily from the diet will have much less impact on your weight loss. This is because, once you have retrained your metabolism, as long as you combine a cheat with protein (your body's new cue not to secrete excess insulin), you will no longer react hormonally to this food in the same way. Instead of storing this 'cheat' food as fat, you remain in a balanced blood-sugar state, and while you may not lose weight at that sitting, you do not have to worry about gaining!

Healthy weight-loss guide – How long do I stay in Phase 1?

My patients lose an average of 18 to 22 pounds over 8 weeks in Phase 1 of **THE NO CRAVE DIET**.

If you are slightly overweight (10–12lb), I would recommend four to six weeks in Phase 1 with adjustment depending on your starting weight and rate of loss.

If you are more overweight (15lb or more), then you will probably need the full eight weeks in Phase 1.

Summary

Meal Timing:

- Three meals per day
- Five to six hours between breakfast and lunch
- Five to six hours between lunch and dinner
- Eleven to twelve hours between dinner and breakfast
- Your aim is not to snack between meals

What you can eat:

- Protein at every meal
- Unlimited – yes, unlimited – salads and most other vegetables
- No grains, rice, pasta or starches
- Two pieces of fruit per day maximum, no bananas
- Limited high-carbohydrate, low-protein foods such as chickpeas and lentils
- Limited portions of dressings and condiments
- None or very limited alcohol (maximum one drink per day)
- Increased fluid levels by drinking more water

Protein at every meal

One of the key features of THE NO CRAVE DIET is protein at each meal: breakfast, lunch and dinner. The actual amount of protein required will depend on how much you weigh. During both Phase 1 and Phase 2 of THE NO CRAVE DIET, your daily protein requirement is calculated as 1 gram of protein per kilogram (2.2 pounds) of body weight.

Example:

If you weigh 90 kilograms you need 90 grams of protein divided between the day's three meals – i.e. about 30 grams per meal – I generally consider the upper limit to be 35 grams per meal, so even if you are over 105kg you should limit yourself to 105 grams of protein per day. Note that your portion of food isn't pure protein, so your actual portion will weigh a lot more, for example 85 grams of chicken provides 20 grams of protein. (see table p.37).

Grams of protein per meal = your weight in kilograms ÷ 3

An easy way to estimate your protein portion

While on **THE NO CRAVE DIET**, we do not want you to worry about weighing food and counting calories. Instead, simply gauge your personal protein size to the size of your hand – let that be your guide at each meal. And it's better to overestimate than underestimate; if you consume a few extra grams of protein at one sitting, it will not cause weight gain; in fact, it will further discourage food cravings later on in the day. So if it is a choice between having a slightly larger or slightly smaller piece of protein, opt for the larger. More importantly, recognise that you need not stress about exact sizes or tedious counting and weighing; we want you to get on and enjoy your meal.

For solid protein sources such as meat, fish, tofu or an omelette, use the easy steps below.

In general most people fall into five protein-size categories, ranging from 15 grams per meal up to 35 grams per meal.

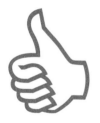

A 'handy' way to judge the correct amount of protein

Step 1: Take your weight in kilograms, then divide by 3 to give you the weight in grams of protein per meal.

Step 2: Using the table below, check this protein portion weight against its protein measurement.

Step 3: Place your hand on a blank piece of paper and draw around the outline.

Step 4: Draw a rectangle on the hand diagram that corresponds to the size of your protein portion.

Step 5: Note how the size of the rectangle relates to your hand.

Step 6: Use your hand whenever you wish to gauge how much protein to eat.

Weight-to-Protein Requirement

Your weight			Grams of protein per meal	Size of protein portion per meal
stones	Lb	kg		
7st 2lb	100	45	15	9cm x 8cm x 2cm
9st 6lb	132	60	20	12cm x 8cm x 2cm
11st 11lb	165	75	25	15cm x 8cm x 2cm
14st 2lb	198	90	30	18cm x 8cm x 2cm
16st 7lb	231	105	35	21cm x 8cm x 2cm

Example: You weigh 75 kilograms.

Step 1: Weight in kilograms divided by 3 = 25. So your protein portion at each meal will be 25 grams.

Step 2: By looking at the table, 25 grams is equivalent to a piece of lean protein (such as chicken) measuring 15cm by 8cm.

Step 3: Draw around your hand.

Step 4: Draw a rectangle measuring 15cm by 8cm.

Step 5: Note that the rectangle is about three-quarters of the size of your hand.

Step 6: At each meal you should eat a protein portion about three-quarters the size of your hand.

How to estimate your protein portion size

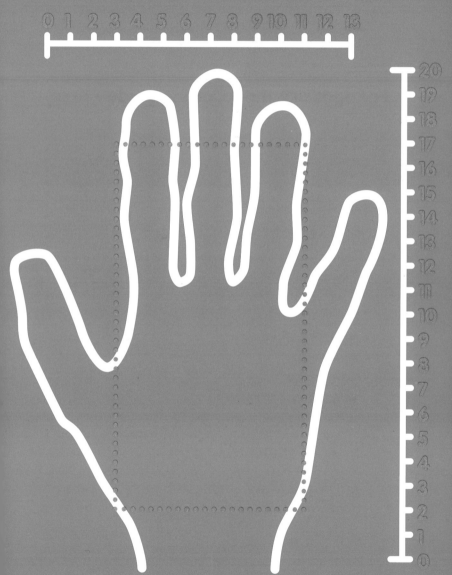

*This diagram is not actual size

Common protein sources are listed below. There must be one protein source from the list below at every single meal. Although there are other foods that contain protein, such as lentils or yogurt, they are not high enough in protein to be counted as ideal protein sources for No-Crave eating. Drink as much water as possible, because the protein forces your body to pass more urine.

• For eggs use the following guide • • • • •

15 grams protein = 2 whole eggs = 4 egg whites

20 grams protein = 3 whole eggs = 6 egg whites

25 grams protein = 4 whole eggs = 8 egg whites

30 grams protein = 5 whole eggs = 10 egg whites

35 grams protein = 6 whole eggs = 12 egg whites

Common protein sources

- Fish
- Chicken or turkey
- Red meat
- Tofu (extra firm, low fat)
- Eggs (5 egg whites to 1 yolk)
- Protein powders – use a whey protein powder with a natural sweetener such as stevia (which, incidentally, also stimulates the immune system), with at least 20 grams of protein and only 3 or 4 grams of carbohydrate per serving
- Protein bars (available from most chemists and some supermarkets) – use bars that are high in protein but low in carbohydrates and fat and contain natural sweeteners
- Low-fat cottage cheese or ricotta cheese

Good protein sources

A good protein source is one that has a good ratio of amino acids specific to the human body, one that is lean or low in saturated fat, and preferably organic. Below is a list of protein sources that fall into this category. The list is in descending order from the best to the worst protein source within this category. It is important to note though, that any protein listed here is of good quality and allowable.

- Egg whites
- Whey protein shakes – with stevia or xylitol
- Fish* (if not organic then wild fish such as tilapia or salmon)
- Turkey*
- Chicken*
- Low-fat tofu
- Low-fat cottage cheese or ricotta cheese
- Back bacon*
- Pork*
- Lean beef*
- Lamb*

*Preferably organic, because many additives increase stress and slow down fat burning.

Egg Whites – the white contains 4 grams of pure protein; the yolk has 3 grams of protein but a large amount of unhealthy fat and cholesterol. Separate the whites from whole eggs or buy cartons of egg white. Add some extra herbs and spices to give the whites more flavour and you will quickly get used to not having all the extra yolk fat. If you find you need the yolk for taste, combine five whites to one yolk.

Whey or Soy Protein Shakes – most are available in small sample sachets so you can try different brands and flavours until you find one you like. Try to find ones with stevia or zylitol as sweeteners. Use water or skimmed milk to make the shake. Adding a little low-fat yoghurt and some berries in a blender makes a tasty protein 'smoothie'.

Poor protein sources

Poor protein sources are those higher in fat or those that have a low proportion of amino acids. These sources should be consumed less frequently (once every two to three weeks or so). Not only are these food sources of lower nutritional value than the good proteins, they are also foods that increase inflammation.

- Nuts in large quantities
- Bacon
- Regular-fat beef
- Sausage
- Deep-fried chicken, pork or beef
- Battered meats

Foods that contain more carbohydrate than protein must be considered carbohydrates and not viewed as protein sources. For instance, legumes, such as lentils and chickpeas, comprise approximately 70 per cent carbohydrate to 30 per cent protein. Try to limit their use. Yogurt is around 75 per cent carbohydrate with only 20 to 25 per cent protein and fat, so think of yogurt as a carbohydrate too.

Protein chart

The first part of this chart compares the amount of protein to fat in each protein source. Some protein sources have a higher fat content than others. Choose leaner protein sources, as they are healthier and cause less craving.

The second part of the chart compares different protein sources by the amount of actual protein they contain. For example, a lean chicken breast weighing about 70 grams will contain about 15 grams of protein, the rest being water and a little fat. On **THE NO CRAVE DIET** we do not want you to start weighing your food. We want to you to use the simple hand-size comparison for your everyday meals. However, by looking at the chart you can gauge which sources provide the most protein. In addition, if you are not sure you are eating the right amount of protein at each meal, a one-time check of the weight of your hand-measured portion will reassure you.

Protein Chart

Protein Source	Protein to Fat Ratio
Egg Whites	All Protein, No Fat
Whole egg	1.3 to 1
Chicken Breast (skinless)	6 to 1
Turkey Breast (skinless)	11 to 1
Salmon (poached)	2 to 1
Tuna (in water)	24 to 1
Trout (grilled)	6 to 1
Beef Steak	2 to 1
Pork Loin	0.7 to 1
Soy (regular)	1 to 1
Soy (low fat)	9 to 1

	Amount you eat to get 15 grams of protein	Amount you eat to get 20 grams of protein	Amount you eat to get 30 grams of protein
Egg Whites	4 – 5 whites	6 whites	8 whites
Tofu (low fat)	85 grams (3 oz)	110 grams (5 oz)	168 grams (6 oz)
Beef (lean)	70 grams (2.5 oz)	85 grams (3 oz)	112 grams (4 oz)
Veal	70 grams (2.5 oz)	85 grams (3 oz)	112 grams (4 oz)
Pork	70 grams (2.5 oz)	85 grams (3 oz)	112 grams (4 oz)
Chicken	70 grams (2.5 oz)	85 grams (3 oz)	112 grams (4 oz)
Turkey	70-84 grams (2.5 to 3 oz)	85 grams (3 oz)	112 grams (4 oz)
Cottage Cheese (low fat)	3/4 cup	1 cup	1 1/2 cups
Ricotta Cheese (low fat)	3/4 cup	1 cup	1 1/2 cups
Cod	80 grams (3 oz)	100 grams (3.5 oz)	126 grams (4.5 oz)
Salmon	80 grams (3 oz)	100 grams (3.5 oz)	126 grams (4.5 oz)
Tuna	80 grams (3 oz)	100 grams (3.5 oz)	126 grams (4.5 oz)
Trout	80 grams (3 oz)	100 grams (3.5 oz)	126 grams (4.5 oz)
Protein Powder	Dependent on the make	Dependent on the make	Dependent on the make
Protein Bar	Dependent on the make	Dependent on the make	Dependent on the make

Carbohydrates
Unlimited salads and most other vegetables

One of the easiest and most enjoyable features of THE **NO CRAVE** DIET is that you can enjoy a wide range of salads and vegetables in unlimited quantities. And we mean unlimited! You really can have as much as you wish. And for those of you who do not believe this to be a particularly exciting prospect, the examples below will show you how these foods can easily replace some of the carbohydrates you will be giving up.

- Mashed cauliflower can replace mashed potato
- Sliced baked carrots or courgettes can replace chips
- Dip celery, instead of nachos, in salsa
- Use cabbage leaves as a wrap for chicken or ground-beef tacos

And because THE **NO CRAVE** DIET includes condiments and dressings, the vegetables and salads in your meal can be healthy and tasty!

Because salads and vegetables are actually carbohydrates, THE **NO CRAVE** DIET is not a 'low-carb' diet. We know you need carbohydrates. You cannot just eat protein alone. Continual protein in high concentration by itself, without any carbohydrate, will stimulate a starvation state called ketosis. This state is unhealthy for the body, particularly the kidneys, so should be avoided. This is why we must add carbohydrates to the meal.

The advantage of salads and vegetables is that they break down very slowly into sugar. They are known as 'complex carbohydrates' because the sugar units are strung together in long, complex chains interspersed with fibre. These long chains take longer to break down into sugar, which reduces hunger and cravings (by causing less of a peak and subsequent drop in blood sugar) but still gives you plenty of energy.

Remember, not all vegetables are 'complex'. For example, potatoes, swedes and turnips contain too much starch and will increase your blood sugar excessively, so avoid these in Phase 1.

Although not the best source of complex carbohydrates, certain vegetables such as carrots and peas are permitted in Phase 1 because they contain beneficial nutrients.

Unlimited carbohydrates – as much as you like!

These may be consumed in unlimited quantities at meals but not between meals:

- Salads and other leafy greens
- All vegetables except potatoes, swedes, corn, yams, turnips and other starchy vegetables
- Cauliflower is unlimited and can be mashed to make an excellent substitute for mashed potato
- Grilled vegetable slices such as courgettes, peppers and carrots make a good substitute for chips

Examples of unlimited carbohydrates:

- Asparagus
- Broccoli
- Green beans
- Cauliflower
- Mushrooms
- Peppers
- Courgettes
- Carrots
- Cabbage
- Cucumber
- Lettuce of any kind
- Tomatoes
- Brussel sprouts
- Snow peas

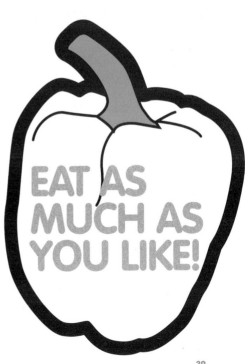

EAT AS MUCH AS YOU LIKE!

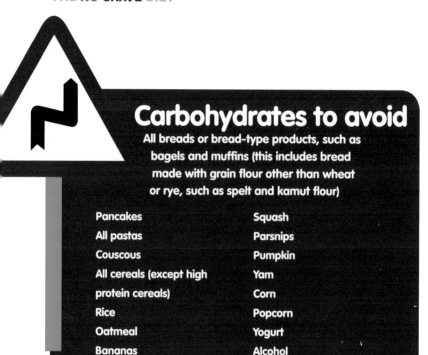

Carbohydrates to avoid

All breads or bread-type products, such as
bagels and muffins (this includes bread
made with grain flour other than wheat
or rye, such as spelt and kamut flour)

Pancakes	Squash
All pastas	Parsnips
Couscous	Pumpkin
All cereals (except high	Yam
protein cereals)	Corn
Rice	Popcorn
Oatmeal	Yogurt
Bananas	Alcohol
Potatoes – sweet and white	Sweets

Vanilla protein powder, soy flour or nut flour can
be used as substitutes for regular flour. They
have essentially no carbohydrate and are high
in protein. They make very nice pancakes,
biscuits and muffins.

Try a protein muffin

The carbohydrates you should avoid

High-sugar carbohydrates need to be cut during Phase 1. All carbohydrates
break down into sugar, so we must select foods that break down more slowly
and produce less total sugar. We must also avoid 'high-sugar' carbohydrates
as these give you persistent hunger and food cravings by causing blood sugar
to peak. Avoiding these types of carbohydrate is a key part of retraining our
metabolism and eliminating cravings and losing weight.

Remember: some of these foods will be reintroduced in Phase 2 of **THE
NO CRAVE DIET** so if they really are on your list of favourite things
you will only be missing them for a short while!

Certain carbohydrates are allowed in limited amounts

A diet based strictly on very 'low-sugar' vegetables and salads can be difficult to follow, so **THE NO CRAVE DIET** makes things easier by allowing a wider variety of carbohydrates even in Phase 1. However, unlike the 'unlimited' carbohydrates, these additional sources are allowed only in limited amounts. These foods are not essential to **THE NO CRAVE DIET** and can be omitted if you wish. They are included to make the diet easier.

Limited high-carbohydrate, low-protein foods such as chickpeas and lentils

Legumes, such as lentils and chickpeas, must be considered carbohydrates because they comprise approximately 70 per cent carbohydrate and 30 per cent protein. They should be avoided or limited to two tablespoons every other day.

- Chickpeas
- Lentils
- Kidney beans
- Lima beans
- Green peas
- Beets
- Refried beans
- Waxy beans
- Split peas
- Pimento beans

How much Carbohydrate can I eat?

Unlimited Salads and vegetables	Phase I	Unlimited
	Phase II	Unlimited
Limited Vegetables and Legumes	Phase I	2 tablespoons every other day
	Phase II	Maximum 1:1 ratio with protein
Fruits	Phase I	2 pieces per day
	Phase II	Maximum 1:1 ratio with protein

The carbohydrate chart on p.42 shows foods in the different carbohydrate categories and the amount of pure carbohydrate they contain. Please note that this chart is not intended to promote the weighing of food; that is not what **THE NO CRAVE DIET** is about. Rather, it allows you to make sensible choices about the foods you eat to better eliminate hunger and craving. Stay within your Phase 1 and Phase 2 food guidelines and choose foods in each category that allow you to eat a greater quantity while minimising carbohydrate intake.

Carbohydrate Chart

Carbohydrates allowed in Phase 1 and Phase 2

Unlimited Salads and Vegetables	Amount you eat to get 10 grams of carbohydrate	Amount you eat to get 30 grams of carbohydrate
Asparagus	20 spears	60 spears
Broccoli (chopped)	8 cups	24 cups
Cabbage	12 cups	unlimited
Carrots	2 large	6 large
Cauliflower	4 cups	10 cups
Cucumber	1 1/2 medium	4 medium
Eggplant	2 cups	6 cups
Lettuce (Boston, Arugala, Leaf)	unlimited	unlimited
Mushrooms	4 cups	12 cups
Onions	3/4 cup	2 1/4 cups
Red Peppers	3/4 large	2 1/4 large
Spinach	unlimited	unlimited
Tomatoes	2 medium	6 medium
Yellow Peppers	2 cups	6 cups

Limited Vegetables/Legumes	Amount you eat to get 10 grams of carbohydrate	Amount you eat to get 30 grams of carbohydrate
Beets	3/4 cup	2 1/4 cup
Green Peas	1/2 cup	1 1/2 cups
Split Peas	1/4 cup	3/4 cup
Black Beans	1/4 cup	3/4 cup
Chick Peas	1/4 cup	3/4 cup
Kidney Beans	1/4 cup	3/4 cup
Lima Beans	1/3 cup	1 cup
Pimentos	1/4 cup	3/4 cup
Refried Beans	1/3 cup	1 cup
Wax Beans	1/4 cup	3/4 cup
White Beans	1/4 cup	3/4 cup

Fruits	Amount you eat to get 10 grams of carbohydrate	Amount you eat to get 30 grams of carbohydrate
Apple	1/2 an apple	1 1/2 apples
Applesauce (unsweetened)	1/3 cup	1 cup
Apricots	3 apricots	9 apricots
Banana	not allowed (too much carbohydrate)	not allowed
Blackberries	1 cup	3 cups
Blueberries	2/3 cup	2 cups
Cantaloupe	1 cup	3 cups
Cherries	1/2 cup	1 1/2 cups
Dates	2 dates	6 dates
Figs	1 fig	3 figs
Grapefruit	1/2 grapefruit	1 1/2 grapefruit
Grapes	2/3 cup	2 cups
Honey Dew Melon	2/3 cup	2 cups
Kiwi	1 kiwi	3 kiwis
Mandarin Orange	1/2 cup	1 1/2 cups
Mango	1/3 mango	1 mango
Nectarine	1 nectarine	3 nectarines
Orange	1 orange	3 oranges
Papaya	1/3 papaya	1 papaya
Peach	1 peach	3 peaches
Pear	1/2 pear	1 1/2 pears
Pineapple	1 cup	3 cups
Plum	1 plum	3 plums
Prunes	2 prunes	6 prunes
Raisins	1/5 cup	1/2 cup
Raspberries	1 cup	3 cups
Strawberries	2 strawberries	6 strawberries
Tangerine	1 tangerines	3 tangerines
Watermelon	1 cup	3 cups

Other foods
Fruit allowed in limited amounts

Fruits need to be limited to a maximum of two pieces of fruit a day. They are actually quite high in sugar and, like carbohydrates, will force the body to secrete insulin. For this reason they should be avoided or consumed in limited amounts: two pieces of fruit per day maximum, and no bananas. Two pieces of fruit includes, for example, one apple and one orange, two grapefruits or one pear and one plum. A cup of sliced fruit or berries is equal to one piece of fruit. It is important to note that one glass of juice is equal to one piece of fruit, but as a source of fruit it is probably the worst choice. The lack of fibre and frequent addition of sweeteners make it much more of a sugar load. Bananas are too high in pure sugar and starch and should be avoided completely.

Dressings and condiments allowed in limited amounts

Dressings and condiments can be used if you wish to add a little extra flavour to your meals. Remember, however, that many of these sauces or toppings can contain a high percentage of fat and sugar. Try to choose ones marked 'low fat' or 'low calorie' as these will generally be healthier and less likely to increase your cravings. If you use them, use them sparingly, perhaps two tablespoons per day.

Cheese and nuts – allowed in limited amounts

Cheese and nuts are allowed only in limited amounts as they are high in fat relative to the protein they contain. The exceptions are low-fat cottage cheese and ricotta cheese, which are excellent protein sources and are included in the protein section above. Treat other cheeses and all nuts like condiments. Sprinkle a few nuts on your salad (try to avoid peanuts due to their inflammatory properties), or add a slice of melted cheese to your vegetables. Remember that these foods are limited and the full 'au gratin' is not an option!

Alcohol – none or limited

The body treats alcohol like a meal of fat and carbohydrate. So besides causing swings in blood sugar and raised insulin it also promotes food cravings.

That desire for a snack after a drink is a combination of low blood sugar and stimulation of the hunger centre. Ideally you should give up all alcohol during Phase 1 of THE NO CRAVE DIET. It is disruptive enough to reduce the effectiveness of the diet at rebalancing your metabolism, lowering your weight and eliminating your cravings.

However, if you really find this aspect of the diet impossible, one drink every other day can be included in Phase 1 (you are not allowed to pool the week's allowance into one on a Saturday night!). Remember that this might increase your cravings, so have it with your meal instead of any dressings, condiments, cheese or nuts.

Drink more water

The change in your diet to include more protein will make you pass more urine. Drinking extra water will help replace this loss of fluid and prevent dehydration, which can act as a stressor and promote hunger and cravings. In addition, water stimulates stretch receptors in the stomach, which will make you feel more full. Keeping your fluids up will also help flush out the toxins released as you start to burn off your fat. Your water can have a slice of lemon (or other citrus fruits) or slices of cucumber, but stay away from juices or cordials, which either contain sugar or artificial sweeteners. Fizzy drinks, including diet drinks, are also to be avoided.

Tea and coffee

Tea and coffee are great beverages to help tide one over until the next meal as they are very low calorie and will not pull you out of fat-burning mode in between meals.

When in herbal or decaf form, they provide important fluids to help hydrate the body and flush fat through. One or two caffeinated drinks a day is permitted, with a small amount (half a teaspoon) of sugar or sugar substitute like Splenda and some milk. Do not overload your beverage with sugar or cream, otherwise further cravings will ensue.

If you wish to drink more than two teas or coffees a day, switch to decaf. Too much caffeine will dehydrate the body and stimulate the release of the stress hormones, which ultimately will increase food cravings and fat storage.

Be careful of all the fancy coffees available today containing chocolate, whipped cream, caramel syrups and sugars. These drinks no longer resemble coffee, but act as liquid dessert. Not only are they high in both sugar and fat, but they will plague you with cravings for sweets and treats for the rest of the day.

No-Crave eating tips
Choose foods that reduce craving

THE **NO CRAVE** DIET is designed to allow you to enjoy a wide range of foods that reduce your hunger and desire to snack. By sticking to these foods you will avoid the pain associated with food cravings.

Choose unsaturated fats

In saturated or 'bad' fats the bonds are single. But the 'good' unsaturated fats have chains in which the bonds between the individual molecules are doubled and are therefore much stronger. They are usually liquid rather than solid at room temperature. Compare olive oil (unsaturated) to lard (saturated). Unsaturated fats are less inflammatory, and impart health benefits such as strengthening hair and skin or promoting a healthy bowel.

Always choose unsaturated fats. They are healthier for you and they are far more effective at letting the brain know that you have eaten and are full. They improve signalling to the satiety centre so you feel satisfied sooner and for longer. The following are examples of unsaturated fats:

- Canola oil
- Olive oil
- Avocado oil
- Soya oil
- Flax oil
- Cottonseed oil

Make it a little spicy

Although excessive flavouring of food can actually promote hunger and overeating (see below), certain herbs and spices on your food can make it taste better and help reduce your cravings. Capsaicin for example, found in red or green chillies, acts on the gut to delay its ability to signal hunger to the brain so you feel full for longer. Eating it early in the morning has actually been shown to reduce overall food consumption during the day (try some red or green chilli pepper in your breakfast egg-white frittata). As an added benefit it also increases your metabolic rate, so you burn more calories.

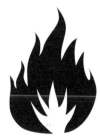

Cinnamon is also a good thing to add to food as it increases your sensitivity to insulin, which will make you feel full faster. It also lowers blood sugar and cholesterol. Try adding some to your protein-flour pancake mix when making your breakfast pancakes (see menu section, page 68).

So go ahead – spice it up!

Avoid foods that increase craving

Changing your diet to include less sugar, starch and saturated fat will automatically reduce your cravings, as these foods actually promote snacking and the desire for more unhealthy foods.

Meals that increase cravings

- Fish and chips
- Pizza
- Chinese food with rice and battered meats
- Lasagne or pasta dishes
- Macaroni and cheese
- Cheese on toast

Snacks that make you crave more

- Twiglets/crisps
- Biscuits/cakes
- Cheese and crackers
- Chicken wings
- Popcorn
- Ice cream

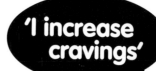

'I increase cravings'

Avoid unhealthy 'reward' food that just encourages more craving

When we eat a piece of food, the body assesses its nutritional content and checks it against our current energy status to determine how much of this food we should eat. With highly palatable sweets or fatty foods, the primary message is that received by the reward centre, which encourages us to eat more regardless of the food's nutritional value or the body's energy needs. The brain's reward system reinforces behaviour that is of no physiological benefit to the body. It is concerned with feeling good, not feeling healthy! Eating these foods reinforces cravings and increases our desire to snack.

Reward foods that increase cravings

- Sugar, chocolate and high-fat foods
- Sweet foods (including those with artificial sweeteners)
- Cakes and pastries
- Crisps
- Ice cream

Not too many different flavours at once!

As mentioned above, some herbs or spices are helpful at reducing cravings, but whilst we do not want our food to be bland and boring, part of our tendency to eat more comes from the reward factor associated with a variety of flavours. The greater the selection of food types, smells and tastes there are at a meal, the more our hunger centre fires, encouraging us to eat more than we need. The all-you-can-eat buffet is probably the most binge-inducing concept on the planet! The extra-large plate, the vast array of tastes, smells and consistencies, and the pressure to really make the most of that 'all-you-can-eat' offer, all contribute to our hunger centre going into overdrive.

So keep your meals simple. Add one or two herbs or spices but don't create a smorgasbord of tastes that will encourage you to keep going back for more. And if you are preparing your own meal, just make enough for what you want to eat.

Avoid most artificial sweeteners

You may think that using an artificial sweetener is a healthy option. However, besides the side effects of these chemicals (some known, some unknown), they are not going to help you lose your cravings. In fact the evidence indicates that they may actually increase them, and they may even make you gain weight, because these so-called low-calorie or no-calorie sweeteners disrupt the body's natural ability to judge the calorific content of a food by its sweetness.

Such sweeteners make our brains believe that we have not really consumed many calories and therefore continue to send out messages from the hunger and craving centres instructing us to eat more. Of course, the foods with artificial sweeteners do actually contain lots of calories in the form of starch or fat, but the body is unable to sense this until much later. So we consume far more calories than we need. Recent research also indicates that artificial sweeteners result in just as much insulin release as real sugar, further explaining the link between weight gain and 'diet' or 'low calorie' foods and drinks.

There are really only two types of sweeteners that are low calorie and do not have a detrimental effect on the body to promote cravings and weight gain. They are named stevia and xylitol. These sweeteners if placed directly on the tongue taste bitter, but when mixed with food create an acceptable level of sweetness. They do not sweeten the food nearly as much as other artificial sweeteners and for this reason they do not confuse the body's sensory system. Sucralose (Splenda), while not as desirable as stevia or xylitol, is the least disruptive of the other sweeteners.

Avoid processed foods

Processed foods often contain extra fat, much of it saturated, as well as simple sugars, refined or bleached flour, and high-fructose corn syrup. From the point of view of your hunger, cravings and weight gain, this is just about as bad as it gets! Not only do these constituents add vast amounts of nutrient-poor calories, they also fail to turn off the hunger centre. Combine that with the 'reward' factor inherently built in to these foods by the manufacturers and you have the ultimate anti-No-Crave meal – lots of calories, very few nutrients and a meal that leaves you unsatisfied and yearning for more. Certainly something to avoid!

Unhealthy processed foods include:

- Canned foods with lots of sodium
- White breads and pastas made with refined white flour
- Packaged snack foods like crisps and cheese snacks
- High-fat foods like cans of ravioli and spaghetti
- Frozen fish fingers and frozen dinners
- Packaged cakes and biscuits
- Microwave meals
- Sugary breakfast cereals
- Processed meats

Avoid foods that cause inflammation

Foods that cause inflammation accentuate cravings by impairing your brain's ability to register the number of calories you have eaten. This prevents it from turning off the hunger message, so these inflammatory foods make you hungrier. They also increase cholesterol production and damage your blood vessels, making them foods to avoid!

Some of the most potent inflammatory chemicals are the trans fats. Not the amount that occurs naturally in animal fats but the extra quantities added to our diets by processed-food manufacturers using hydrogenated plant oils. This practice has led to a tremendous rise in our intake of trans fats.

They are found predominantly in vegetable shortenings, some margarines, packaged or processed foods such as biscuits, crackers, snack foods, cakes, crisps, breakfast cereals and salad dressings, and in fried 'fast foods'. Besides their effect on your weight and cravings, the inflammation caused in your blood vessels markedly increases your risk of heart disease. So you should completely avoid processed foods containing high levels of trans fats.

Other foods known to produce inflammation (albeit at lower levels) are the deadly nightshades, which include potato, aubergine (eggplant) and tomatoes, some animal products such as red meat and dairy foods, and nuts, particularly peanuts. Of course, we are not suggesting you cut out all of these foods, but it would be advisable to minimise their intake, or avoid combining too many of them at one sitting.

Foods that cause inflammation – avoid large quantities

- Cheeses, especially the aged ones
- Red meat
- Peanuts
- Highly processed foods, especially cold meats (hams, salami, etc.)
- Foods high in white refined sugar (white bread, cakes, scones, etc.)
- Corn oil
- Margarine
- Nightshade foods – aubergine, tomato and potato

Foods that reduce inflammation

Eating certain foods will actually decrease the amount of inflammation in your body and reduce cravings. Foods containing omega-3 essential fatty acids, such as salmon, mackerel, tuna or tofu, are ideal. In addition these foods are also rich in protein, which we know has many other benefits for weight loss and food cravings.

Berries such as blueberries and strawberries contain powerful antioxidant phytochemicals that decrease inflammation, help prevent heart disease and provide beneficial fibre at the same time.

Spicing up your food with turmeric or ginger greatly reduces inflammatory load. These spices possess powerful ingredients to directly inhibit the production of inflammatory substances, as well as protecting surrounding tissues from generating inflammation. Bring on the curry!

Foods that reduce inflammation – these are good for you!

- Fish – especially cold-water fish such as salmon and mackerel
- Walnuts
- Pecans
- Soy/tofu

- Dark green vegetables such as spinach and broccoli
- Canola oil
- Pumpkin seeds
- Berries
- Red onion
- Unpeeled apple
- Grapefruit

Meal planning on THE **NO CRAVE** DIET

Here are a few tips that will make the early stages of your diet even easier, helping to further reduce hunger and cravings as the effects of THE **NO CRAVE** DIET kick in.

No-Crave your home and workplace

Clean out your cupboards and your fridge by removing snacks and crave-inducing foods. Any bouts of craving will be much easier to resist if the nearest biscuit is twenty minutes away at the local supermarket. Make sure you have something healthy available in the event of a craving 'emergency'. This has to be something that will have minimal impact on your No-Crave Diet. I recommend some vegetable sticks (celery, broccoli, cauliflower, peppers are best), a quarter of a protein bar (keep the rest in the freezer), a spoonful or two of cottage cheese, a few nuts (walnuts may work best to reduce cravings) or make up a small protein shake. Remember, however, THE **NO CRAVE** DIET works best with no snacking between meals!

The importance of protein at breakfast

The word breakfast comes from 'breaking the fast'. If you extend the fast, either by skipping breakfast or eating a meal higher in carbohydrate than protein, you will encourage fat storage. First thing in the morning, because your blood sugars are low, you need to wake up the metabolism and stabilise your fat-storing hormones with the necessary amount of protein (one gram of protein per kilogram of body weight divided by three).

By eating protein at breakfast you will decrease hunger hormones and inhibit fat storage for the next eight hours. The protein sets your metabolic controls for most of your day, orienting it to burn up the calories you eat at each meal and to burn your fat stores in between each meal. So banish food cravings and jump-start your day with a power-packed protein breakfast.

Help! I'm so hungry!

During the first week on **THE NO CRAVE DIET**, your body may experience some side effects – increased hunger, light-headedness, irritability and slight nausea. Do not be alarmed! Your brain is rebelling against your attempt to get your hunger centre under control. The feelings are normal and will rapidly subside after a few days on **THE NO CRAVE DIET**.

Your body is designed to burn fat between meals so that you have sufficient energy without getting hungry, but until you retrain your metabolism through Phase 1 you will not have access to these stores. You will keep relying on sugar, which as soon as levels get low will trigger your hunger. Your brain's hunger centre, which has been running your life, will protest over the first few days, often making you feel very hungry between meals. But have faith: if you stick with the diet this will stop within a week.

If you are finding hunger pangs, nausea or light-headedness too much to cope with then try increasing the amount of protein you have at each meal, say from 20 to 25 grams, and drink more water between meals. If this still does not work try eating a small protein snack between meals. Snacks are not strictly permitted on **THE NO CRAVE DIET** as they pull you out of fat-burning mode but, for the first few days, a very small protein snack – for example, one third of a protein bar or a protein shake or two tablespoons of cottage cheese – can help get you through to the next meal.

Although we don't want you feeling faint and weak, remember it is OK to be hungry sometimes. We have grown up with the thought that hunger is bad – a habit we have to break. In most cases hunger does not mean you have no energy supplies left. Take a look at when your hunger hits – if you only have one hour to go to the next meal, have a glass of water and wait the hour. However, if you are faint, nauseated or can't concentrate, then have a small snack.

Another possible cause of increased hunger and nausea is the natural detoxification process that begins when you start **THE NO CRAVE DIET**. As soon as you start eating healthy, nutritious food on a consistent basis and cut out the fried, fatty and sugary foods, your liver no longer has to work at dealing with these food toxins. It can therefore increase its normal workload, detoxifying potent chemicals from the environment that are stored in the body. Like any detoxification processes this may have slight side effects, including hunger and nausea. For 10 emergency No-Crave measures, see p.119.

Tips for a meal out

Here are some useful tips to help reduce cravings during a meal. These are particularly helpful if you are planning to eat out, for example a work lunch or an evening with friends.

- Eat fibre or a little 'good' fat before your meal
- Drink a couple of glasses of water before your meal
- Eat your salad or vegetables first
- Ask for vegetable sticks instead of bread

Eating a little fibre before your meal or before you go out to eat is very effective. You can have a few sticks of celery, carrot or broccoli or there are a few types of fibre drinks you can use. The first and most soluble is inulin fibre (see Supplement section). One teaspoon of this before a meal will not only decrease hunger and activate the satiety centre in the brain, it will also slow down the delivery of sugar into the bloodstream, thereby decreasing insulin release and the storage of food as fat. Other types of fibre that can be taken in either capsule or powder form are de-fatted (fat and oil removed) flax and/or borage.

Another alternative is to consume a little good (healthy) fat. We should stick to these healthy fats in order to minimise the small quantity of bad (saturated) fats that we inevitably consume in foods like salad dressings, cheese, nuts and the fat within some of our protein sources. So, as a pre-meal hunger-reducing snack the healthiest – and incidentally the most effective – is an omega-3 fat (fish or flax oils) in capsule or liquid form. This will stimulate the satiety messengers in the gut (especially CCK) making you less hungry initially and full sooner. If you don't have these, a few unsalted walnuts or an omega-oil enriched dip (with a few vegetable sticks) is an excellent alternative.

If you forget the fibre or fat or suddenly find yourself in a situation where you do not have a chance to plan ahead, start your meal with a couple of glasses of water and then order your salad first. That way you will feel full once the main course arrives, allowing you to eat less and leave the potatoes and rice if they arrive by mistake.

At a restaurant the bread bowl usually arrives early. Ask your waiter to bring vegetable sticks instead.

The importance of plate size

Here are three easy ways to make things easier for yourself:

■ Use smaller plates

■ Never eat from a container

■ Make or order only what you want

It is well known that over the past twenty years portion sizes have grown dramatically. Most of us were always told to finish everything on our plate, and not to waste our food. This may have been OK when our plate sizes were much smaller. Today the physical size of the average dinner plate has increased by almost 50 per cent. Unfortunately we are not just putting the same amount of food on the larger plate, we are managing to fill the larger plate with a bigger portion. In addition, we use side plates for vegetables and salads, the foods that should be taking up most of the space on our dinner plate. Of course, this leaves more room for rice, potatoes or pasta on the main plate.

Restaurants and fast-food outlets are mostly to blame as they promote even bigger portions, often for the same price, to outdo their competitors. Our consumer attitude is so highly tuned to the concept of a 'good deal' that this marketing ploy is irresistible. Bigger must be better value. Combine that with our inherent disapproval at leaving food behind – a trait impressed upon us as children – and we have a recipe for calorie disaster.

So use smaller plates at home or, if eating out, ask for the meal on a small plate. You will be surprised how little you notice the change in portion size.

Secondly, never eat directly from a container; always transfer the food onto a plate. This way you set out how much you want to eat and have some idea of how much you have eaten.

Thirdly, make or order only what you wish to eat. If you want only one chicken breast, do not be tempted to order the 'half-chicken special'; it contains more food than you need and probably has a side order of potatoes or pasta.

Note: The exception to this last rule would be at home when you are making a batch of healthy meals such as protein chilli, chicken stir-fry or egg frittata for the week.

Avoid distractions at meal times

Always sit down to eat your meal and avoid concurrent activities such as watching television. Evidence shows that individuals who stand or walk while eating or consume their meal in front of the TV eat far more than they normally would. Such distractions appear to counteract our satiety cues.

Chapter 2: Recipes
BREAKFASTS

With each of the following breakfast recipes, you can have the following:

**175ml/6oz glass
of skimmed milk**

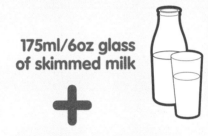

+

**Decaffeinated coffee or
herbal tea with low-fat milk
and/or sugar substitute**

Egg No-McMuffins
Berries for Breakfast!
Smoked Salmon Scramble with Hash Browns
Salsa Frittata with Sausages
Breakfast Bahama-Mama
Eggs Benny with Hollandaise Sauce
Low-Carb Strawberry Smoothie
Ham and Cheese Crêpes
High-Protein Pancakes
High-Protein Muffins

Egg No-McMuffins

Makes 12 muffins

12 slices lean streaky bacon
6 medium-size free range eggs, beaten
180ml/6fl oz milk
½ red or green pepper, cored and finely chopped (optional)
½ medium onion, finely chopped (optional)
1tsp ground black pepper
125g/4½oz reduced fat Cheddar cheese, grated

1. Preheat oven to 180°C, Gas 4.

2. Line 12 muffin tins with large squares of non-stick baking parchment so they stick up like crowns and spray lightly with a vegetable-oil cooking spray to prevent sticking.

3. On the bottom of each tin, place a single slice of bacon, so that it sticks above the tin, or curl the bacon around the inside of the tin.

4. In a bowl, whisk together the egg, milk and black pepper and, if you like, add in the peppers and onion.

5. Pour the liquid mixture into each of the foil tin liners, filling each one to the top.

6. Sprinkle the top of each with grated cheese.

7. Bake for 20 to 25 minutes until the filling is firm and the cheese melted.

8. Let them stand for 5 minutes to cool, then remove the 'muffins' from the tins and serve.

Tip: you can wrap these in cling film and refrigerate for a few days, then microwave them on high for about 30 seconds to reheat.

Berries for Breakfast!

Makes 2 servings

500ml/18fl oz soy or skimmed milk

300g/10oz fresh blueberries, raspberries, strawberries or a mixture of all three

½ banana

1 x 125g carton natural yogurt

50g/2oz whey or soy protein isolate powder

40g/1 ½oz ground flaxseeds (optional)

1. In a blender, blend together the milk, fruit and yogurt until smooth.

2. Add in the protein powder and flaxseeds and blend until thoroughly mixed.

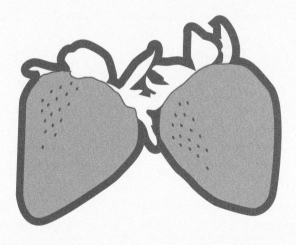

Smoked Salmon Scramble with Hash Browns

Makes 2 servings

4 egg whites

1 whole egg

2tbsp skimmed milk

¼tsp ground black pepper

1tsp rapeseed oil or low-fat vegetable cooking spray

50g/2oz smoked salmon sliced or chopped

1tbsp chopped fresh dill

For the hash browns:

1tbsp rapeseed oil

4 slices lean back bacon, diced

½ onion, chopped finely

1 small courgette, chopped

4–5 cauliflower florets, chopped

2 egg whites, lightly beaten

Sea salt and ground black pepper to taste

To make the Smoked Salmon Scramble

1. In a bowl, whisk together the egg whites, the egg, the milk and the pepper.

2. In a non-stick frying pan, heat the oil (or spray with low-fat vegetable-based cooking spray) over a medium-low heat and add the egg mixture.

3. Gently stir the eggs until they begin to set. Add the smoked salmon and continue to cook until the eggs are completely set.

4. Sprinkle with the dill and serve with the Hash Browns.

Tip: try using diced shrimp, crabmeat or cooked lobster (canned or pre-packaged, drained) in this recipe.

To make the Hash Browns

1. In a large non-stick frying pan, heat the rapeseed oil and cook the bacon and onion until they just start to brown.

2. Add the courgettes and cauliflower; cover the pan and cook over a medium-low heat until the vegetables are tender.

3. Add a bit more oil if required to brown the vegetables and stir occasionally.

4. Once the vegetables have softened, add your eggs and season to taste.

5. Continue cooking over a medium-low heat until the bottom is browned. Flip and brown the other side and divide into 2 servings.

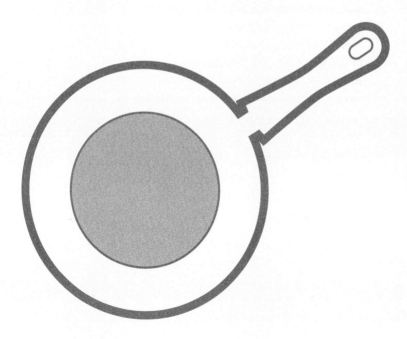

Salsa Frittata with Sausages ··········

Makes 2 servings

1tsp rapeseed oil

4 spring onions, trimmed and chopped

½ medium red and/or green pepper, cored and chopped

1 small courgette, chopped

1 finely chopped jalapeno pepper – seeds removed (optional)

A dash of dried oregano, sea salt and ground black pepper to taste

2 free range eggs, beaten

125g/4½oz low-fat cottage or ricotta cheese (NB – UK ricotta not low fat)

4 tbsp skimmed milk

25g/1oz mild grated Cheddar cheese

2–4 large slices of tomato

2tbsp salsa dip (mild, medium or hot – your choice!)

2 sausages (see cooking tip below)

1. Pre-heat the grill.

2. In an ovenproof or cast-iron saucepan, heat the oil over a medium-low heat on the hob and sauté the vegetables until wilted and soft, about 5 minutes. If you want your frittata spicy, add your jalapeno pepper at this stage and sauté with the other vegetables.

3. Stir in your seasonings and continue cooking for another 2 minutes. Remove from heat and reserve.

4. In a bowl, whisk together the egg, cottage or ricotta cheese and milk until well mixed and pour over the vegetables in your pan.

5. Cook the mixture over a medium-low heat until the bottom has set, but it's still liquid on top.

6. Remove from the heat, sprinkle the grated cheese over the top and place under the grill for 2 to 3 minutes until the cheese has melted and the top has set.

7. Remove, divide into 2 portions. Arrange the tomato slices on two plates and serve each frittata on top with the salsa dip.

> Tip: In the microwave, cook the sausages for about 4 to 5 minutes on high, on a plate lined with paper towel to absorb any of the fat. Try using different types of sausages such as Cumberland, sage and onion, honey-garlic or spicy Italian.
>
> If you want to spice this up even more, add in half a cup of diced, cooked, spicy Italian sausage to the egg mixture. Cook your sausage in the microwave in advance and add it to the vegetables before you add your egg mixture.

Breakfast Bahama-Mama

Makes 2 servings

8 strawberries
1 mango
600ml/1 pint water
4tbsp pina colada mix (see below for a recipe)
2tbsp whey or soy protein isolate powder
2tsp flax oil (optional)
8 ice cubes
For the sugarless pina colada mix:
2tbsp coconut milk or cream
6tbsp unsweetened fresh pineapple juice
1 small scoop of vanilla, low-sugar frozen yogurt
1 sachet or 1tbsp Splenda

1. In a blender, process all the ingredients.

2. Put on your bathing suit. Lounge by the pool.

Sugarless Pina Colada Mix

1. Combine everything in blender and add to the Bahama-Mama recipe above.

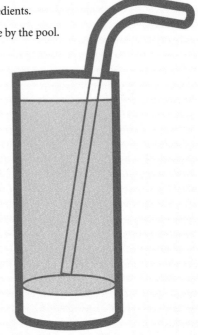

Eggs Benny with Hollandaise Sauce

Makes 2 servings

4 slices lean back bacon
A pinch of salt
2tbsp white wine vinegar
1 free range egg + 3 egg whites
For the hollandaise sauce:
125g/4½oz unsalted butter
2tbsp fresh lemon juice
¼tsp sea salt
4 large free range egg yolks
1 dash Tabasco sauce

1. For the hollandaise sauce, microwave the butter, 1tbsp lemon juice and salt in a medium bowl (covered with cling film) on high until the butter melts, about 1 minute. Whisk to cool slightly.

2. Whisk in the egg yolks until blended.

3. Microwave (covered) on medium power for 30 seconds and whisk until blended. Repeat this step twice.

4. Whisk in the remaining lemon juice and the Tabasco sauce. Keep warm.

5. Dry fry the bacon in a non-stick pan or the microwave and set aside on four warmed plates.

6. Fill another non-stick pan three-quarters full of water, add a pinch of salt and the vinegar and bring to a boil. Reduce the heat to a simmer and place in four poaching rings.

7. Mix together the egg and whites and pour into the poaching rings and simmer for 2½ minutes over a medium heat.

8. Remove a poached egg, place it on top of the bacon and top with the hollandaise sauce.

Low-Carb Strawberry Smoothie.....

Makes 2 servings

250g/9oz strawberries

180g/6½oz silken tofu

500ml/18fl oz skimmed milk

2tsp Splenda

2 scoops (40g/1½oz) whey or soy protein isolate powder

1. Combine everything in a blender and top with a fresh strawberry.

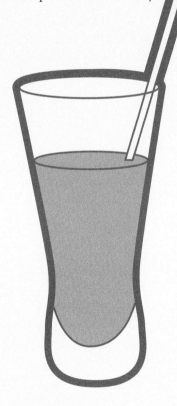

Ham and Cheese Crêpes

Makes 2 servings

For the filling:

125g/4½oz chopped cooked ham or cooked pork loin

60g/2¼oz grated Gruyere or Emmenthal cheese

Sea salt and pepper to taste

For the crêpes:

50g/2oz vanilla protein powder (or protein flour substitute)

½tsp sea salt

4 free range eggs, lightly beaten

25g/1oz butter, melted and slightly cooled

350ml/12fl oz soy milk

1tbsp chopped fresh parsley

1tbsp chopped fresh or dried rosemary

2tbsp chopped fresh chives

¼tsp freshly ground pepper

1. Combine the chopped ham or pork and cheese and set aside.

2. Mix the protein powder and salt in a bowl and create a well in the middle. Add the soy milk, eggs and butter and whisk until thoroughly combined.

3. Strain through a sieve, pressing against any lumps until you have a smooth batter. Add your herbs, salt and pepper to the batter at this point, and combine well.

4. Spray some low-fat cooking spray into a pan and heat over a medium-high heat.

5. Using a ladle pour about 2tbsp of batter in the middle of the pan, moving the pan around to evenly coat the bottom.

6. Cook for about 60 seconds, then flip and cook for 15 seconds more.

7. Add 2tbsp of the filling to each crêpe and fold over onto itself.

High-Protein Pancakes

Makes 2 servings

40g/1½oz finely ground almonds
40g/1½oz vanilla protein powder
1¼tsp baking powder
¼tsp sea salt
4tbsp of Splenda
3 free range egg whites
25g/1oz butter, melted
250ml/9fl oz semi-skimmed or skimmed milk

1. In a bowl, mix the ground almonds, vanilla protein powder (or other protein powder), baking powder, salt and Splenda together.

2. In a separate bowl, mix the melted butter, milk and egg whites together.

3. Slowly combine the wet mixture with the flour mixture, folding and stirring evenly until the mixture is smooth with no lumps.

4. Preheat a frying pan on a medium-high heat.

5. Add a little butter, oil or non-stick spray oil to the pan.

6. Using a ladle pour about 4tbsp of pancake batter per pancake into the pan and swirl to coat the base evenly. Once bubbles appear on top of the pancake, flip over and cook the other side.

Note: these can be made up in batches and frozen individually. They can then be toasted like frozen waffles. Berries, lemon juice and Splenda mixed together make a great syrup alternative.

High-Protein Muffins

Makes 8-12 muffins

115g/4oz butter, softened
25g/1oz Splenda
1tbsp vanilla extract
150g/5oz vanilla protein powder
300g/12oz nut flour
5tsp baking powder
250ml/9floz milk
225g/8oz fresh or frozen blueberries

1. Preheat the oven to 190°C, Gas 5.

2. Thoroughly mix together the butter, Splenda, vanilla extract, protein powder, nut flour, baking powder and milk.

3. Add the blueberries last (and gently, with a spoon, to keep them whole).

4. Grease 8 sections of a large muffin tin, or 12 regular-size muffin sections and pour in the batter until half full.

5. Cook the muffins until you can stick a knife in and it comes out clean or dry.

LUNCHES

With each of the following lunch suggestions, you can have the following:

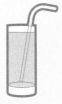

175ml/6fl oz glass of sugar-free vegetable juice cocktail or tomato juice

Decaffeinated coffee or herbal tea with low-fat milk and/or sugar substitute

Asian Tossed Veggie Salad with Chicken and Lemon-Lime Sauce

Peasant Soup

Spinach, Bacon and Mushroom Salad with Dijon Dressing

Hot and Sour Soup

Thai Seafood Soup

Chickpea and Tuna Salad

Caesar Salad with Grilled Salmon or Chicken

Roasted Middle Eastern Vegetables with Tzatziki

French Vegetarian Cassoulet

'Club Sandwich' Salad

Asian Tossed Veggie Salad with Chicken and Lemon-Lime Sauce

Makes 2 servings

A good handful each of cooked broccoli, cauliflower, snow peas or mangetouts, courgettes

1 small head green cabbage or spring greens, shredded finely

A handful of cherry tomatoes

1 cooked chicken breast, about 150g/5oz, sliced

1–2tbsp sesame seeds

For the lemon-lime sauce:

2tsp rapeseed oil

1tbsp sesame oil (or more rapeseed oil)

2½tsp white-wine vinegar

½tsp lemon juice

½tsp lime juice

1tsp water

1 pinch freshly chopped ginger

1. Make the lemon-lime sauce first. Place the sauce ingredients together in a screw-top jar with a tight-fitting lid and shake vigorously until well combined

2. Steam your vegetables ahead of time. Cut up a few pieces of broccoli, cauliflower, mangetouts and courgettes and place them in a bowl covered with about 2.5cm/1 inch of water. Microwave on high for 4 to 5 minutes until just tender, but still crunchy.

3. Toss your mixed greens, tomatoes and steamed vegetables together in a bowl. Place the sliced chicken breast on top of the vegetable mix.

4. Drizzle the dressing over the top of the greens and vegetables and sprinkle the sesame seeds on top.

Tip: try using a poached salmon fillet with this salad instead of the chicken breast.

Peasant Soup

Makes 6-8 servings

3 leeks, white ends only
4 carrots, peeled
3 parsnips, peeled
6 cloves garlic, chopped fine
125g/4½oz unsalted butter, or lower-fat butter substitute
1 litre/18fl oz chicken or vegetable stock
12 plum tomatoes, cut in 2.5cm/1inch chunks
500g/1lb 2oz chopped cooked chicken, turkey or firm tofu
2–3tbsp flat-leaf parsley, roughly chopped
12 large basil leaves
1½tsp dried tarragon
1½tsp freshly ground pepper
1tsp nutmeg
Sea salt to taste
125g/4½oz grated Cheddar

1. Cut the white ends off the leeks, leaving about 2.5cm/1 inch of green. Remove the outer skin, slice in half lengthwise and rinse thoroughly then chop into small pieces.

2. Cut the carrots and parsnips into small diced pieces and add to the leeks. Add the garlic to this vegetable mixture.

3. Melt the butter or lower fat butter substitute in a large pot over a low heat. Add the vegetables and cook covered for about 10 minutes, stirring occasionally until the vegetables are wilted.

4. Add the stock, stir and continue cooking covered for another 10 minutes. Add the tomatoes, chicken (or turkey or tofu) and seasonings, stir, cover and cook for another 15 minutes over a medium heat.

5. Remove the cover and simmer on a low heat for 30 minutes.

6. Adjust the seasonings, and serve in a bowl with the grated cheese on top.

Spinach, Bacon and Mushroom Salad with Dijon Dressing

Makes 2-4 servings

500g/1lb 2oz baby leaf spinach

250g/9oz raw mushrooms, thinly sliced

½ red onion, thinly sliced

5 hard-boiled eggs, whites only, coarsely chopped

5 strips lean bacon, fried crisp, drained and crumbled

For the Dijon Dressing:

120ml/4fl oz rape seed or olive oil

½tsp toasted sesame oil

1tsp Splenda or sugar substitute

3tbsp freshly squeezed lemon juice

½tsp Dijon mustard

Sea salt and freshly ground black pepper to taste

1. Wash and spin-dry the spinach and discard any stems.

2. Toss the spinach, mushrooms, onion, egg whites and crumbled bacon in a bowl.

3. To make the dressing, place all the ingredients in a screw-top jar and shake vigorously. Adjust seasonings if required. Pour over the spinach salad and toss until all the leaves are coated. Serve immediately.

Hot and Sour Soup

Makes 6-8 servings

500g/1lb 2oz skinless, boneless chicken breasts (about 4)

2.8 litres/5 pints water

Small wine glass of rice wine, sake or dry white wine

8 thin slices of fresh ginger

8 spring onions, ends trimmed, cut into 2.5cm/1in pieces

250g pack firm tofu, drained, cut into strips 2.5cm/1in long and 1 cm/½in thick

250g/9 oz raw mushrooms, sliced thin (or try oyster or shitake mushrooms)

2 medium leeks, white part only, cut in julienne strips

1 large free range egg white, lightly beaten with 2tbsp water

Seasonings:

 4½tbsp Worcestershire sauce

3tbsp low-salt soy sauce

3tbsp minced fresh ginger

¾tsp freshly ground black pepper

1tsp sesame oil

1. Cut the chicken breasts into thin julienne strips. Place the chicken pieces in a large pot with the water, rice wine or sake, ginger and onions and bring to a boil. Simmer on a low heat, partially covered, and cook for about 30 mimutes.

2. Remove the ginger and green onion pieces from the broth with a slotted spoon and skim the surface of any fat.

3. Add the tofu, mushrooms and leeks to the chicken and heat again to boil for 2 to 3 minutes.

4. Add the seasonings and stir on a low heat for about 5 to 10 minutes. Taste and adjust seasonings.

5. Remove the soup from the heat and slowly add the beaten egg white and water mixture, pouring it in a thin stream in a circular path around the pot, and then stir it in the same direction with a large spoon to make the egg into wispy streams.

6. Serve immediately.

Tip: this soup is delicious the next day, heated through on low heat (or microwave a single serving on medium heat for 3 minutes, stir and then heat again on medium-high for 2 minutes).

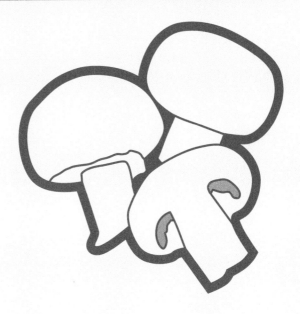

Thai Seafood Soup

Makes 6-8 servings

150g/5oz white fish fillet (cod, haddock, coley, sole, tilapia)
8 large prawns, shelled and de-veined
3 crab sticks, cut in 1cm/1 in chunks
8 large mussels, scrubbed
250g/9oz squid, thawed if frozen
125g/4oz mushrooms, quartered if large
1 stick of lemon grass
2.5cm/1in fresh ginger root
100ml/3½fl oz fresh lime juice
1.2l/2 pints water
5tbsp Thai fish sauce
3tbsp chilli paste
2 hot red chilli peppers, sliced thinly (optional if you like it hot!)
A handful of fresh bean sprouts
Basil or coriander leaves, to serve

1. Prepare the seafood. Cut the fish fillets into 1cm/½in chunks and set aside. Set all the shellfish aside.

2. Smash the end of the lemon grass with the flat end of a knife (or mallet) and then slice into 1cm/1in pieces. Peel the ginger root and slice into thin rounds.

3. Bring the water to the boil in a large pot, turn to a medium-high heat and add the lemon grass pieces, the ginger root rounds and 2tbsp of the lime juice. Cook for 2 minutes. Add the fish sauce, chilli paste and cook for another 2 to 3 minutes.

4. Remove the lemon grass pieces and ginger root rounds with a slotted spoon and discard.

5. Cook the fish and seafood in the following order: add the fish chunks and cook for 2 minutes; add the prawns, crab sticks and mussels and cook for another 2 minutes until the mussels open (throw away any that do not open).

6. Add the mushrooms to the soup. Add remaining lime juice, and adjust your seasonings. If you want it spicier, dice the sliced chilli peppers to the soup.

7. Serve in a bowl and garnish with raw bean sprouts, basil leaves or coriander leaves, roughly chopped.

Chickpea and Tuna Salad

Makes 2 servings

1 x 200g can of light tuna, drained and flaked
½ avocado, halved and stoned and cut in chunks
½ x 400g can of chickpeas, drained
½ x medium red onion, chopped
1 fresh pepper, red, green or yellow, diced
For the dressing:
1tbsp olive oil
1tbsp fresh lemon juice
¼tsp dried oregano
Sea salt and pepper to taste

1. Toss the tuna, avocado, chickpeas, onion and bell pepper in a bowl.

2. Combine the dressing ingredients in a jar and shake vigorously until mixed, and then drizzle over the salad.

Tip: use this as a side dish or salad with one of the dinner menu selections.

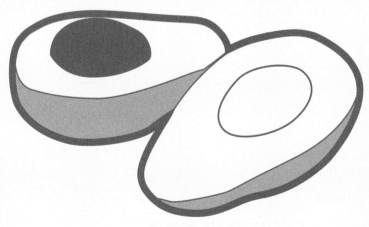

Caesar Salad with Grilled Salmon or Chicken

Makes 2 servings

1 small cos lettuce, shredded

2tbsp Caesar salad dressing (see below for recipe)

1tbsp freshly grated Parmesan cheese

1 x 250g/9oz skinless, boneless chicken breast or salmon fillet, grilled and sliced (see Dinner menus for grilling recipes)

For the salad dressing:

1 free range egg yolk

3tbsp red-wine vinegar

1tbsp Splenda

1tbsp chopped fresh garlic

Sea salt and freshly ground black pepper, to taste

250ml/9fl oz olive oil

4tbsp freshly grated Parmesan cheese

For the salad:

1. Toss the lettuce in a large salad bowl with the Caesar salad dressing and Parmesan cheese.

2. Slice the chicken or salmon fillet on the diagonal and place on top of the salad.

For the dressing:

1. Whizz the egg yolk, vinegar, Splenda, garlic, salt and pepper in a blender to combine then, with the motor running, slowly dribble the oil in a steady stream until thick and creamy.

2. Add in the Parmesan cheese, taste and adjust seasonings and blend again. Chill until ready to use.

> Tip: this garlic dressing is excellent drizzled over a platter of fresh, raw vegetables or can be used as a dip.

Roasted Middle Eastern Vegetables with Tzatziki

Makes 2-4 servings

4tbsp rape seed or olive oil

1½tsp sea salt

1tbsp finely chopped fresh ginger root

¾tsp ground cinnamon

¾tsp ground coriander

½tsp ground cumin

½tsp dried chilli flakes

1 medium head broccoli, broken into florets

1 medium cauliflower, broken into florets

1 red onion, halved and thickly sliced

1 carrot, cut into 1cm/½in slices

1 small aubergine, cut into 2.5cm/1in chunks

1 x 400g can of chickpeas, drained and rinsed

125g/4½oz cooked chicken or tofu

Vegetable spray

3tbsp chopped fresh coriander

For tzatziki:

250g/9 oz natural low-fat yogurt

½ cucumber, halved, seeded and diced

1tsp chopped fresh garlic

½tbsp olive oil

1½tbsp white wine vinegar

2tbsp chopped fresh dill

3tbsp chopped fresh mint

¼tsp sea salt

1. Preheat the oven to 220°C, Gas 7.

2. Mix together the oil and spices in a large bowl then toss in the vegetables.

3. Spray a small roasting pan with the vegetable spray, tip in the coated vegetables in a single layer, cover loosely with foil and cook for 20 minutes.

4. Remove from the oven, stir the vegetables and cook, uncovered, for another 20 minutes.

5. Stir in the chickpeas, tofu or chicken and roast uncovered until the vegetables are slightly browned and tender (approximately 10 minutes).

6. Sprinkle with the coriander and serve with the tzatziki below.

For tzatziki:

1. Combine all the ingredients above into a blender and process until smooth. Chill until ready to use.

2. Serve as a dipping sauce for the vegetables.

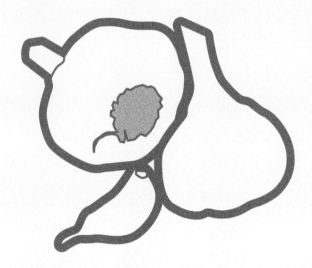

French Vegetarian Cassoulet

Makes 6-8 servings

200g/7oz dried white beans, e.g. haricot or cannellini

1 Spanish onion, halved

1.2 litres/2 pints vegetable stock

4 whole cloves of garlic

2 sprigs of fresh parsley

1 sprig of fresh thyme

1 bay leaf

2tbsp olive oil

2 carrots, cut into 1cm/½in rounds

½ acorn squash, cut into 2.5cm/1in chunks

250g/9oz celeriac, cut into 1cm/½in pieces

Sea salt and freshly ground pepper to taste

2tbsp olive oil

1 red onion, chopped

1 celery stick, chopped

150g/5oz Brussels sprouts, ends trimmed, cut in half

250g/9oz mushrooms, coarsely chopped

250g/9fl oz dry white wine

3tbsp tomato purée

1tbsp fresh rosemary, chopped

1tsp each dried oregano and thyme

1. Place the beans in a large bowl, cover with water and soak overnight. Drain and reserve the beans.

2. Place the beans, Spanish onion, vegetable stock, garlic cloves, parsley, thyme and bay leaf in a large pot and bring to a boil. Cover and simmer for 90 minutes or until the beans are done.

3. Strain the cooking liquid into a large bowl and reserve. Remove the onion, parsley, thyme and bay leaf from the beans and set the beans aside.

4. Preheat the oven to 220°C, Gas 7.

5. Toss the carrots, squash and celery root with the 2tbsp oil and add salt and pepper to taste. Spread the coated vegetables in an even layer on a foil-lined baking sheet and roast for 25 minutes, until brown but still firm. Remove from oven and set aside.

6. Reduce oven to 180°C, Gas 4. In a large pot, heat 2tbsp oil over a medium-high heat and add the red onion, celery, Brussels sprouts and mushrooms, and stir occasionally for 10 minutes until the vegetables are softer.

7. Stir in the wine, tomato paste, rosemary, oregano and thyme and a bit more salt and pepper to taste, and cook for 2 minutes longer. Now stir in the reserved beans.

8. Spread half of the bean mixture on the bottom of a 4 litre oven proof casserole. Top with the roasted vegetables, and then the remainder of the bean mixture.

9. Pour in the reserved cooking liquid and bake uncovered for another 90 minutes.

Tip: try adding mild Italian sausage, chunks of pork loin, or even pieces of cooked lamb to this dish for a meatier version.

'Club Sandwich' Salad

Makes 2-4 servings

1 large head of iceberg lettuce, torn into bite-sized pieces
2 large tomatoes, cut into wedges
1 spring onion, chopped
2 free range eggs, hard-boiled, whites only chopped
10 lean rashers streaky bacon, cooked and crumbled
250g/9oz cooked turkey or chicken, cubed
250ml/9fl oz 'blender mayo' (see recipe below)
Sea salt and pepper to taste
For blender mayo:
1 free range egg
¼tsp sea salt
½tsp dry mustard or 1tsp Dijon mustard
250ml/9fl oz rape seed or olive oil
1½tbsp fresh lemon juice
1tbsp boiling water
Sea salt to taste

1. In a large bowl, combine and toss together the lettuce, tomatoes, green onion, egg whites, bacon and turkey or chicken. Add the salad dressing, salt and pepper to taste.

For blender mayo:

1. Place the egg, salt, mustard and a quarter of the oil in a blender. With the blades still running, slowly add the remaining oil in a steady, thin stream.

2. Add the lemon juice and 1tbsp of boiling water.

3. Adjust seasoning to taste, and chill until needed.

Dinners

With each of the following dinners, you can have the following:

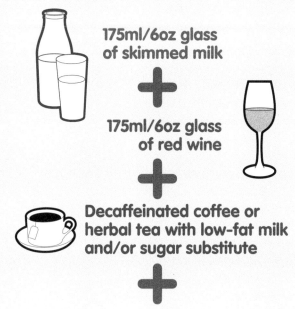

**175ml/6oz glass
of skimmed milk**

+

**175ml/6oz glass
of red wine**

+

**Decaffeinated coffee or
herbal tea with low-fat milk
and/or sugar substitute**

+

Meat Loaf with Green Beans and Cauliflower Mashed 'Potatoes'
Lemon Chicken Breasts with Zucchini and Carrots
Grilled Thai Salmon with Snow Peas
Pork Tenderloin with Berry Fruit Glaze and Roast Vegetables
Herb Roasted Chicken with Spinach Mushrooms
Steak with Balsamic Vinaigrette and Rosemary Beans
Sole Packets with Steamed Vegetables
Rosemary Garlic Lamb Chops with Stuffed Peppers
Butternut Squash Arrabbiata
Ratatouille

Meat Loaf with Green Beans and Cauliflower Mashed 'Potatoes'

Makes 6-8 servings

90g/3¼ oz textured vegetable protein

1 onion, chopped fine

2 free range eggs, slightly beaten

500g/1lb 2oz lean minced beef

500g/1lb 2oz minced turkey or chicken

2tbsp Worcestershire sauce

1½tsp dry mustard powder

1½tsp sea salt

½tsp ground black pepper

176ml/6fl oz skimmed or soy milk

For the cauliflower mashed 'potatoes' (makes 2 servings):

1 medium-size cauliflower, trimmed of stalks and chopped

1tbsp butter

1tbsp reduced-fat crème fraiche

Sea salt and ground black pepper to taste

5 strips cooked bacon, crumbled (optional)

Handful green beans to serve

1. Preheat the oven to 180°C, Gas 4 and spray a loaf pan or casserole dish (roughly 25cm x 15cm) with low fat vegetable-oil cooking spray.

2. Combine all the ingredients together in a large bowl, using your clean hands to mix it together.

3. Put the mixture in the loaf pan and bake for 45 minutes to 1 hour.

Tip: refrigerate the meat loaf in the pan overnight and the next day remove it from the pan, leaving behind any fat. Slice it up and serve it cold with one of the salad suggestions from the lunch menus.

Steamed green beans:

1. Take a handful of green beans and cut the ends off. Wash thoroughly, place in a steamer basket and steam for 5 to 10 minutes. If you have a microwave, steam them in a microwave bowl for 3 to 5 minutes on high. They should be cooked through, but still crunchy.

> **Tip:** sprinkle your beans with one of the following: feta cheese, almond slices, fresh mint or pine nuts.

Cauliflower mashed 'potatoes':

1. Steam or microwave the cauliflower until it's soft enough to mash, and strain well.

2. Add the butter and crème fraiche, salt and pepper to taste, and mash until you have the consistency of mashed potatoes. Stir in crumbled bacon if desired.

> **Tip:** use 1tbsp of garlic butter instead of regular low-fat butter or sauté 1tsp of chopped garlic in your butter for 2 to 3 minutes over a medium-low heat to infuse your butter with the garlic taste, and then add to the mashed 'potatoes'.

Lemon Chicken Breasts
with Zucchini and Carrots

Makes 2-4 servings

4x 150g/5oz boneless, skinless chicken breasts
120ml/4fl oz freshly squeezed lemon juice
4tbsp olive oil
2tbsp cracked or roughly ground black peppercorns
Low-fat vegetable cooking spray
For zucchini and carrots:
4 medium carrots, cut into thin julienned sticks
2 medium courgettes, cut into thin julienned into sticks
2tbsp butter
2tbsp chopped fresh parsley
Sea salt and freshly ground black pepper to taste

1. Spear the chicken breasts several times with a sharp pointed knife or sharp fork and place in a small bowl large enough to hold the chicken, or in a heavy plastic food bag.

2. Mix the lemon juice, olive oil and pepper together and pour over the chicken. Twist to seal or cover and marinate for 20 to 30 minutes.

3. Remove the chicken from the marinade and, if using a grill or barbecue, spray with the non-stick cooking spray and sear the chicken breasts for 1 minute on each side, then move off the direct heat and cook for 5 to 7 minutes longer until done. You could also bake the breasts in a hot oven for 3 to 4 minutes each side until done.

Tip: double the recipe and keep the remaining cooked chicken breasts in the refrigerator; serve sliced on top of one of the lunch salad suggestions.

For zucchini and carrots:

1. Place the carrot sticks on the bottom of a steamer basket and place the courgettes sticks on top. Place the steamer in a pot over 2.5cm/1 inch of salted water, and steam for 10 to 12 minutes until tender but not soft. Or you could use a microwave steamer – microwave on high for 5 minutes, then let stand for 2 to 3 minutes.

2. Drain and place in a serving bowl with salt and pepper to taste.

3. Melt the butter in a saucepan or microwave, stir in the chopped parsley and pour over top.

> **Tip:** instead of using butter, drizzle the vegetables with lemon juice and grind some freshly ground pepper on top.

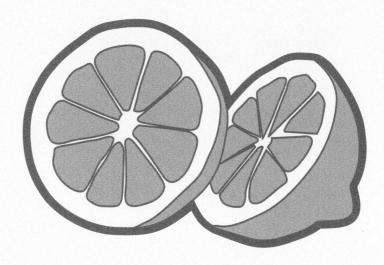

Grilled Thai Salmon with Snow Peas

Makes 4 servings

4 salmon fillets or salmon steaks, about 120g/4 oz each

1tbsp chopped garlic

2tbsp low salt soy sauce

1tsp ground pepper

1tbsp Splenda or sugar substitute

1tbsp rape seed oil

For the Thai sauce:

250ml/fl oz white or rice vinegar

25g/1oz Splenda or sugar substitute

2 tbsp low salt soy sauce

2 tbsp chilli-garlic sauce

1 tbsp chopped garlic

Handful green beans to serve

1. Place the salmon in a glass pie plate.

2. Combine the remaining ingredients in a bowl and pour over the salmon, turning to cover them completely. Marinate for 30 minutes.

3. Grill the salmon for 5 to 7 minutes each side, depending on thickness, until done.

4. To make the Thai sauce: Combine the vinegar and sugar substitute in a saucepan over a medium-high heat until dissolved. Add the soy sauce, stir and cook over a medium-high heat for 6 to 8 minutes until slightly reduced. Remove from the heat and stir in the chilli-garlic sauce and the extra chopped garlic.

5. Pour the Thai sauce over the top of the salmon and serve.

Tip: cook extra salmon fillets and serve with a tossed green salad for lunch. Pour the sauce cold over the top as a salad dressing.

For mangetouts:

1. Take a handful of mangetouts and cut the ends off. Wash thoroughly, place in a steamer basket and steam for 3 to 5 minutes. If you have a microwave steamer, steam them for 1 or 2 minutes on high. They should be cooked through, but still crunchy.

Tip: line a plate with lettuce leaves, place your salmon fillet on top, pour your Thai sauce over it and sprinkle with chopped red pepper and coriander leaves; serve your mangetouts on the side.

Tip: this recipe also works really well with grilled chicken breasts.

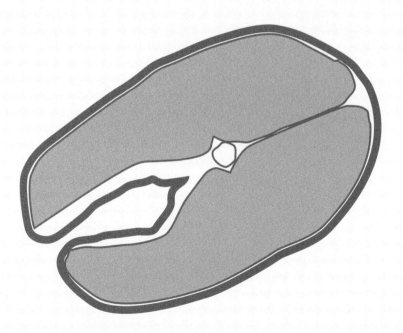

Pork Tenderloin with Berry Fruit Glaze and Roast Vegetables

Makes 4 servings

1.8kg/4lb boneless pork loin

4 tbsp rapeseed oil

250ml/9fl oz vegetable stock

Berry fruit glaze
(recipe below)

1tbsp chopped garlic

2tbsp fresh or dried rosemary

Sea salt and ground
black pepper to taste

For berry fruit glaze:

5–6 tbsp low-sugar
red berried jam or
redcurrant jelly

3tbsp Splenda or
sugar substitute

2tbsp port

4tbsp low-sugar cranberry
or grape juice

For roast vegetables:

4 tbsp olive oil

2tbsp coarse sea salt

1tsp each of oregano
and thyme

1tbsp fresh rosemary,
chopped

1 medium cauliflower,
stems trimmed and
broken into florets

1 head of broccoli,
stems trimmed and
broken into florets

1 each red onion and carrot,
cut in 1cm/½in slices

1 x 400g can
chickpeas, drained

1. Preheat the oven to 180°C, Gas 4.

2. Pour the oil all over the roast and rub it in with your hands, then place it fat side up in a shallow roasting pan.

3. Pour the vegetable stock in the bottom of the pan.

4. Pour the berry fruit glaze over top of the roast.

5. Top with the chopped garlic, rosemary, salt and pepper.

6. Roast for 1½ to 2 hours until the internal temperature reads 70°C.

7. Allow to stand for 15 minutes before carving.

Berry fruit glaze:

1. In a saucepan on a low heat, melt the jam or jelly, Splenda or sugar-substitute and stir until thoroughly combined.

2. Stir in the port and berry juice and heat through to combine until the jelly is dissolved. Pour over the pork for roasting.

Tip: serve cold slices of this roast pork with a spinach salad for lunch.

Roast vegetables:

1. Preheat the oven to 220°C, Gas 7.

2. Mix together the salt and herbs in a big bowl and set aside.

3. Toss all the vegetables with the olive oil and then toss with the salt and herbs mixture to coat.

4. Roast for 20 minutes covered, then remove cover, stir, and roast uncovered for another 10 minutes.

5. Add the chickpeas, stir again and roast another 10 minutes until the vegetables are tender.

Herb Roasted Chicken with Spinach Mushrooms

Makes 2-4 servings

1 chicken about
1.5–1.8kg /3–4lb

Sea salt and freshly ground
black pepper to taste

250ml/9fl oz chicken
or vegetable stock

3tbsp butter

For the herb marinade:

120ml/4fl oz olive oil

350ml/12fl oz rapeseed oil

7 cloves of garlic

4 sprigs of fresh rosemary

4 sprigs of fresh thyme

Freshly ground black
pepper to taste

For the spinach mushrooms:

250g pack leaf
spinach, washed

Sea salt to taste

8 large mushrooms

1tbsp chopped garlic

2tbsp rapeseed or olive oil

1. Place all the marinade ingredients in a bowl and mix well. Place the chicken in the bowl and coat it with the marinade sauce. Cover the bowl and marinate overnight, turning the chicken occasionally.

2. Preheat the oven to 220°C, Gas 7 and prepare your barbecue by turning it to high.

3. Season the chicken and sear it on the barbecue for about 3 minutes on all sides.

4. Transfer the seared chicken to a roasting pan and roast in the oven for about 45 minutes until done.

5. Remove the chicken from the pan and set aside covered in aluminium foil to keep warm.

6. Pour off any excess chicken fat from the roasting pan and add the vegetable or chicken stock. Cook over a high heat for 1 or 2 minutes, scraping any browned bits.

7. Add the butter to the juices, adjust your seasonings and cook for an additional minute over a high heat. Strain the juices into a gravy jug.

8. Carve the chicken and served topped with the pan juices.

Spinach mushrooms:

1. Cook the spinach in a large pan with a little water and salt to taste, until just tender, then drain well, squeezing out excess water and chop coarsely.

2. Remove the stems from the mushrooms, coarsely chop the stems and set both aside.

3. Heat the oil in a pan and sauté the chopped garlic over a low heat for 1 or 2 minutes (don't let the garlic brown).

4. Add the mushroom stems to the garlic-infused oil over a medium-low heat until done, about 3 minutes. Remove from the pan, mix with the spinach and set aside.

5. Sauté the mushroom caps for 4 to 5 minutes, as above (add a bit more oil if required).

6. Divide the spinach/chopped mushroom mixture onto each of the mushroom caps and serve.

Steak with Balsamic Vinaigrette and Rosemary Beans

Makes 2 servings

600g/1lb 4oz rump or sirloin steak, in one piece
250ml/9fl oz balsamic vinegar
2tbsp chopped Spanish onion
Sea salt and freshly ground black pepper to taste
For the rosemary beans:
2 x 400g cans of cannellini beans
5–6tbsp chicken or vegetable stock
4 cloves of garlic, finely chopped
1tbsp of fresh chopped rosemary or ½tbsp dried
Sea salt and freshly ground black pepper to taste

1. Trim any excess fat from the meat.

2. Place in a bowl or large plastic food bag with the vinegar and onion and marinate for 30 minutes. Preheat the grill.

3. Drain, season with salt and pepper to taste and place on the grill pan and cook 5 to 7 minutes for medium-rare if the steak is thin, or 8 to 10 minutes if it's thicker. Cook longer if you prefer it more well done.

4. Remove from the heat, cover with foil and let stand for 5 minutes.

5. Slice on the diagonal against the grain and serve with the beans.

6. To prepare the rosemary beans: Drain but don't rinse the beans. Place the beans in a saucepan with the stock, garlic and rosemary and cook over a medium heat for about 5 minutes, until warmed through. Drain, add salt and pepper to taste and serve.

Tip: serve cold slices of this beef with a spinach salad for lunch. The beans are also good cold as a side dish.

Sole Packets with Steamed Vegetables

Makes 4 servings

4 pieces of aluminium foil big enough to wrap the fillets
Low-fat vegetable spray
1 small carrot, grated
1 stick celery, finely chopped
½ small onion, finely chopped
4 sole fillets, skinned, about 150g/5oz each
1 lemon, juice freshly squeezed
4tbsp fresh dill, chopped
Sea salt and ground black pepper to taste
Lemon wedges, to serve

1. Preheat the oven to 220°C, Gas 7.

2. Lay the aluminium foil sheets flat and spray with the low-fat vegetable spray.

3. In a bowl, mix together the carrot, celery and onion. Take half of this mixture and divide it between the 4 pieces of foil.

4. Place the sole fillets on each bed of vegetables and top with the remaining vegetables then drizzle the lemon juice over top.

5. Top with chopped fresh dill and add salt and freshly ground pepper to taste.

6. Fold over the ends and twist to seal to create sealed parcels. Bake on a baking sheet for 10 to 15 minutes, depending on the thickness of the fillet.

7. Open the top (watch the steam!) of each parcel to serve with a lemon wedge.

Tip: try this cooking method with cod, bass, red snapper, tilapia or other fresh fish fillets. Also try adding different vegetables to the mixture: asparagus tips, green beans, zucchini or snow peas, for example.

Rosemary Garlic Lamb Chops .... with Stuffed Peppers

Makes 4 servings

4 lamb chops, about 200g/7oz each

½tbsp rapeseed oil

1tbsp fresh rosemary or ½tbsp dried, chopped

4 cloves of garlic, crushed

Sea salt and freshly ground black pepper to taste

For stuffed peppers:

4 whole peppers, red, yellow or green

2tsp olive oil

2tbsp balsamic vinegar

1 large clove of garlic, crushed

500g pack plum tomatoes, quartered, seeded and coarsely chopped

125g/4½oz firm mozzarella cheese, grated

Fresh basil leaves from 2–3 sprigs, cut in strips

Sea salt and freshly ground black pepper to taste

1. Preheat the oven to 180°C, Gas 4 and line a baking sheet with aluminium foil.

2. Place the lamb chops in a bowl and coat with the oil.

3. Top each chop with the rosemary and garlic.

4. Heat a non-stick pan over a medium-high heat and add the chops. Cook for 2 minutes each side until browned. Add salt and pepper to taste.

5. Transfer the chops to the baking sheet and cook in the oven for another 10–15 minutes to finish.

Stuffed peppers:

1. Preheat the oven to 190°C, Gas 5

2. Cut the tops off the bell peppers, and carefully scoop out the ribs and seeds.

3. Very carefully, cut off the 'bumpy' bottoms of the peppers, just enough so that they can stand flat on their ends. Be careful not to cut too deeply or the filling will run out of the bottom.

4. Combine the remaining ingredients in a bowl until well mixed.

5. Stuff each pepper with the filling.

6. 'Sit' each pepper in a casserole dish, sprayed with a non-stick vegetable spray, and bake until the bell peppers are done, about 40 to 45 minutes.

Tip: try using the Ratatouille or the Arrabbiata sauce (see recipes following) as an alternative filling for these peppers.

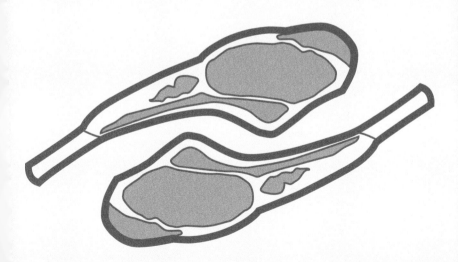

Butternut Squash Arrabbiata

Makes 2 servings

4tbsp rapeseed oil

4–6 cloves of garlic, crushed

1 large onion, diced

500g/1lb 2oz lean minced beef, veal or pork (or a combination)

2 x 200g cans chopped tomatoes

1 green pepper, cored, seeded and diced

1 red pepper, cored, seeded and diced

12–15 mushrooms, sliced

1½tsp dried oregano

1½tsp dried basil

Sea salt and ground black pepper to taste

1 butternut or acorn squash

2tsp butter

Freshly grated Parmesan cheese, to serve

Sea salt and ground black pepper to taste

1. Heat the oil in a large frying pan or wok over a medium heat, and gently sauté the garlic for 2 to 3 minutes (don't let it brown).

2. Add the onion and sauté over a low heat until softened, about 10 minutes.

3. Add the meat, stirring to break up, and toss with the garlic and onion, then cook over a medium heat until the meat is cooked through, about 10 minutes.

4. In another pot, add your tomatoes, green and red peppers and mushrooms and simmer over a low heat. Add your meat, onion and garlic mixture to this when it's done.

5. Add your seasonings and let simmer for an hour over a low heat, slightly covered.

6. Meanwhile, halve the butternut or acorn squash. Prick all over with a fork and spread a teaspoon of butter on each half. Sprinkle with salt and pepper.

7. Place each half in a bowl with a little water and cover tightly with cling film. Microwave on high for 8 to 10 minutes until done.

8. Adjust your seasonings to the sauce and place a large heaped spoonful of the meat sauce into each half of the cooked squash.

9. Top with grated Parmesan cheese and freshly ground pepper.

Tip: try combining low-fat ground chicken or turkey with the ground beef to reduce the fat in this recipe. Also, try using different types of squashes to vary the 'look' of this meal. Replace the peppers with zucchini if you like.

Ratatouille

Makes 6-8 servings

160ml/5½fl oz olive oil

4 small aubergines, cut into 2.5cm/1in cubes

7tsp sea salt

2 red onions

7 medium courgettes, cut into 5cm/2in strips

4 whole peppers, red, yellow or green, cored, seeded and sliced into 1cm/½in strips

2tbsp garlic, crushed

3 x 400g cans of diced plum tomatoes, drained

1 x 140g can of tomato purée

4tbsp fresh Italian flat-leaf parsley, roughly chopped

4tbsp fresh dill

2tsp dried basil

2tsp dried oregano

Sea salt and freshly ground black pepper to taste

425g/15oz chopped cooked chicken or tofu

1. Preheat the oven to 200°C, Gas 6 and line a roasting pan with aluminium foil.

2. Pour in half the olive oil, add the aubergines, sprinkle with the salt and toss to coat.

3. Cover the pan and bake for 30 minutes until the aubergine is done, but not mushy. Uncover and set aside to cool.

4. In a large frying pan or wok, heat the remaining oil and sauté the onions, courgettes, peppers and garlic over a medium heat until wilted and tender, about 20 minutes.

5. Add the tomatoes, tomato purée, fresh and dried herbs and salt and pepper to taste. Stir well and continue to simmer for 10 more minutes, stirring occasionally.

6. Add the aubergine and chicken or tofu to the tomato mixture and simmer for another 10 minutes.

7. Adjust seasonings and serve immediately.

> **Tip:** try using this Ratatouille as a filling for the Stuffed Peppers recipe above.

Chapter 3: Strategies for Phase 1
10 daily No-Crave temptation therapies

THE **NO CRAVE** DIET incorporates not just dietary changes but other ways to stave off cravings. No man is an island – and no diet is an island. Trying to change just one thing in your life, the food you eat, is akin to surrounding yourself with water. When life on the island gets tough there is nowhere else to go. So build some bridges to the mainland and use them when you feel your personal 'diet island' is getting a little too claustrophobic. Even just knowing those bridges are there will make your diet that much easier.

Lifestyle changes do not have to be extreme. They are simple techniques aimed at reducing the stress associated with dieting and food cravings, supporting yourself and changing the way you use snacking to deal with other issues. Not only will this be important as you progress through the diet, but in the long term it will prevent you slipping back into old habits at times of stress or emotional upheaval.

1. Remove temptation!

One of the first things you should do when starting THE **NO CRAVE** DIET is to spring-clean your kitchen, fridge and larder. Whilst the diet, supplements and other therapies will eliminate your cravings, this may take a few days and, during that time, having your favourite snack staring back at you every time you open the fridge is not going to make life any easier. The harder a snack is to obtain the less likely you are to eat it! If you are craving a few crisps you are much more likely to give in if they are sitting on the shelf by the television rather than at the corner shop, a ten-minute walk away in the rain! Of course, if you live with other people who may not be sharing your commitment to a healthy lifestyle, getting them to help you is important. If they refuse to get rid of all snack food, ask them to keep only snacks they like and you don't, and keep those away from the areas where you will be working or cooking.

Once you have removed temptation, replace the unhealthy foods now in the bin with healthier ones that fit your No-Crave Diet plan. While I do not encourage any snacking, it may be useful to have something available in the first week or so in case of emergencies. I recommend some vegetable sticks (celery, broccoli, cauliflower and peppers are best), a quarter of a protein bar (keep the rest in the freezer), a spoonful or two of cottage cheese, a few nuts (walnuts may work best to reduce cravings), or make up a small protein shake.

You also need to remove temptations at work, so that packet of crisps or sweets in your desk drawer needs to go!

2. Simple stress-management techniques

Stress is one of the most significant factors in diet failure. It has an uncanny ability to promote hunger and food cravings while providing an 'excuse' to drop off your diet. You tell yourself you are justified in having that tasty snack because you are 'stressed', and that once the stress is gone you'll be right back on track. Unfortunately it never works like that. Stress is so prevalent in most of our lives that the one-off snack inevitably becomes a regular event, the snacking itself making you feel worse, causing more stress and causing you to crave another snack, and pretty soon you've blown your diet. Now that's stressful!

So, instead of reaching for the tub of ice cream, try one of the simple stress-management techniques outlined below. They are easy to perform, take very little time and are surprisingly effective in any stressful circumstance. When combined with a regular programme to reduce your overall chronic stress they provide a healthy alternative to the biscuit barrel.

Instant stress relievers

- Deep breaths – take five slow, deep breaths with your eyes shut (if practical). This is a quick version of the deep-breathing exercise below and will work best once you have practised the full exercise.

- Visualisation – write down the name of one of your 'relaxation places' and spend a few minutes visualising it. (Further details are explained in the visualisation exercise on page 165.)

- Three-minute seated meditation.

- Put on some of your favourite music, close your eyes and listen.

- Play with your pet if you have one – studies show this to be an extremely effective stress reducer.

Deep breathing can become part of your daily routine. You may wish to deep breathe for five minutes in the morning before you leave for work, when you get home or just before bed. In addition, the technique can be used during the day to alleviate stress and anxiety-related craving. In this latter situation you will have to modify the exercise. For example, closing your eyes may not always be practical (or safe!). You may not be in a comfortable spot and only have time for a few breaths. However, once familiar with the relaxation that deep breathing instils, that is all it will take to defuse your stress whether in traffic, a supermarket line or a board meeting.

1. Find a quiet, comfortable place to sit. Turn off distractions such as radio, television or telephone. Rest your hands on your knees or clasp them lightly in your lap.

2. Close your eyes and let your mind be aware that it is time to relax. Repeating a word such as 'calm' or 'peace' a few times may help at this point.

3. Become aware of your breathing. Rather than it being an automatic activity occurring in the background, concentrate on each breath. Feel the air entering and leaving your lungs over four or five breaths.

4. Breathe in through your nose and out through your mouth to start with, and then, as your breathing deepens and you start to relax, in and out through your nose.

5. Try to breathe more deeply, using your diaphragm and abdomen rather than just your lungs.

6. As your breaths get deeper, pause very briefly between inhaling and exhaling, being aware at that point of the oxygen and energy filling your body.

7. Then pause slightly between exhaling and inhaling, allowing your body to completely relax at that very moment.

8. Try counting during inhalation and exhalation. Start with a count of three on breathing in and five on breathing out. If this feels comfortable increase the exhalation count a little at first and then the inhalation count.

9. As you breathe, feel yourself relaxing, sinking deeper into the chair.

10. Continue for as long as you wish.

11. On completion of the exercise open your eyes, return your breathing towards normal, and stretch. Bring your arms out straight then raise them slowly above your head, allowing them to touch before bringing them back to your side. Do this three times.

12. Get up slowly and in stages.

Note: During the exercise, do not hyperventilate. If you begin to feel dizzy or sick, open your eyes and stop the exercise. Concentrate on something else until your breathing returns to normal and any untoward sensations have passed.

For more stress-management techniques, including visualisation, see page 163.

Reducing Your Daily Stress

Besides using the simple techniques above to cope with sudden stress-induced cravings, a regular lifestyle change to reduce your overall stress levels is important. Incorporate daily deep breathing, meditation or visualisation exercises. Consider bodywork techniques including yoga, Tai Chi, massage, aromatherapy or reflexology.

Lifestyle changes

1. No multi-tasking

Do not multi-task. Although you may think this is a time-efficient way to go about things, you will rapidly become overloaded. The more stimuli you impose upon yourself, the greater the activity of your stress glands. Keep your tasks or jobs simple; that means one at a time, and do them well. When you are finished move on to the next.

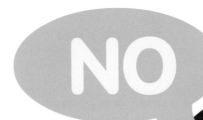

2. Learn to say 'No'

People often have a problem saying no
to others for fear of hurting or upsetting them. They end
up saying yes to everything, taking on too much and hurting
themselves. Learn what your boundaries are, and how much you
can handle. Once you reach that limit, do not take on any more. Others will
understand, for they themselves are on overload, otherwise they would not be
asking for your help.

3. Avoid known stressors

If there are certain parts of your day where you know you will encounter
stressors, try to alter your pattern. For instance, if you get upset in traffic try not
to leave the house at rush hour. Get up a little earlier so you can miss the traffic
– and possibly go for a workout before you start work. Then you can leave the
office sooner and miss the traffic on the way home. If you can't avoid the traffic,
then prepare yourself for it. Bring some soothing music to listen to, or a tape of
something you want to learn. At least then if you are sitting in traffic, you can
enjoy yourself.

4. Don't set unrealistic goals

Many of us want to do everything and do it as quickly as possible. We are
impatient and our society has programmed us to expect results straight away,
whether that be in health care, career advancement, or via high-speed Internet!
Our failure to achieve goals is a major stressor. Reset your goals to be attainable,
and attainable within realistic time frames.

5. Positive affirmation

Wake up and look in the mirror and take note of one positive thing a day. If
you see something you don't like, then look away for now. Don't focus on the
negative. Try to find something positive in everything, however hard that may
seem. The actual process of looking for 'good' is calming – and finding it will
improve your mood and outlook.

Massage

By reducing stress and increasing your feel-good brain hormones, dopamine and serotonin, massage makes you more relaxed, happier and it decreases your hunger-centre activity. This leads to less stress and less craving.

Massage therapy is defined as the treatment of disease or injury through the manual manipulation of body tissues. Massage is employed for the relief of pain and spasm, to induce relaxation, to stretch and break down scarring and adhesions, and to increase circulation and metabolism. Massage promotes the resorption and metabolism of toxins and the residua of inflammation. The basic movements include effleurage, petrissage, friction, tapotement, and vibration.

The relaxation benefits of massage therapy are not just subjective – massage has been shown to decrease both noradrenaline and cortisol levels in the blood, urine and saliva. That wonderful feeling you get at the end of a massage is not just from lying down quietly for a period of time. There is a significant therapeutic effect from receiving regular massage therapy, which clearly goes far beyond simple musculoskeletal pain relief.

Safety: Contraindications are few. Following acute injury or a severe flare-up of an existing injury, or in the presence of an open wound, local massage would not be advisable in that area. However, distant massage or massage therapy performed on other parts of the body is advisable to help increase the effects of the immune system and decrease inflammatory mediators, and cortisol levels. In order to receive these benefits, massage can be performed anywhere on the body. It is avoided in certain cancers to avoid promoting spread.

Simple massage techniques can also be practised at home to help relieve stress.

1. Use a massaging shower-head, which augments the benefits of superficial heat from the water.

2. Move a simple wooden roller-type massager back and forth across the neck, back or feet.

3. Use commercial electric massagers, with or without heat.

4. Have a partner apply slow, gentle, finger, thumb or hand pressure.

Aromatherapy

Aromatic healing oils can be used during a therapeutic massage. These essential oils are absorbed both through inhalation and through the skin during a treatment. Throughout the massage, lymphatic drainage, muscle releases and spinal pressures are applied to target the nervous system, and affect every organ and muscle of the body. Each oil has a different effect, ranging from detoxification and relaxation to increasing energy levels.

Essential aromatherapy oils for relaxation and stress relief are:

- Amber
- Bergamot
- Camphor
- Cedarwood
- Lavender
- Poppy
- Ylang-ylang

And there are several ways you can use essential oils:

- Diffuser – a small metal bowl heated by a candle
- A few drops in a warm bath
- In a massage oil
- A few drops in a facecloth or sponge in the shower
- As a perfume

3. Setting your 'diet commandments'

Diet commandments are phrases and thoughts that are designed to help inspire you during **THE NO CRAVE DIET**. They act as reminders and motivators when you have a craving, and keep you feeling positive on your diet.

Your personal list of diet commandments should be read every morning. It is an easy way to start each day with a reminder and motivator as to why you are taking charge of your diet and your health. Your commandments should also be kept near you at all times during the day (in your desk at work, or in your purse) so that when you have a food craving, you can simply pull your list out, reread it and understand why you should not give in to that food craving.

To begin your diet commandment list, start out by identifying and writing down personal reasons why you want to lose weight and what it means to you. This may be as simple as wanting more energy and reducing your blood-cholesterol levels, or you may want to provide a positive role model for your children. You might be trying to overcome a long love–hate relationship with food and your body image. Also write down what it would mean to you to be slimmer, healthier, energetic and happy. Identify with what that feels like. At the same time write down what it feels like to be overweight, tired and unhealthy. Identify with those feelings, and understand why you no longer want to experience them, and that you are making the conscious decision to replace those physical and emotional feelings with positive healthy, happy and balanced ones. Start each day by reading these commandments: your personal reasons and goals and why you want to follow your programme. In time, your body will 'hear' this message, and it will be easier to follow the diet. Just like when you first start exercising, you may dislike getting up, putting on your running shoes and getting out the door. But as soon as it becomes routine your body responds positively. Words work in the same way. Keep reading them and your body will crave **THE NO CRAVE DIET**.

Write down small reminders for yourself that reinforce the no-cheat mechanisms. For instance, if you crave a biscuit, instead of mindlessly grabbing for the biscuit, think about it. Think about the last time you ate one. Most likely you had about thirty seconds of satisfaction followed by several hours of hypoglycaemia, further food cravings, guilt and other self-defeating thought processes. Write down and reread this reminder every time you crave – that thirty seconds of satisfaction is simply not worth twenty-four hours of feeling mentally and physically unwell.

In your commandment list, you should also have a reminder of what to do if you have cheated. Firstly, recognise it was one cheat, and stop it there. No one ever gained twenty pounds or failed a diet from one cheat. Many people have gained weight or failed at the weight-loss process from one cheat leading to another and another. Many of my patients feel that if they cheat once in the day they have blown the whole day, so they continue to eat and eat, telling themselves that they will restart tomorrow. Do not do this – start right now. It was only one cheat. Let this diet commandment guide you away from the biscuit barrel.

Your diet commandment list will act like your own personal counsellor, motivator and reminder. They might include some of the following examples:

- I want to be healthier and have more energy to spend with my family
- I want to lower my cholesterol and blood pressure and decrease my risk of cardiovascular disease
- I do not want my children to grow up with an overweight, sick or unhealthy role model
- I want to fit into the myriad of clothes hanging in my closet that are too tight right now
- I want to get this weight off once and for all and feel confident in myself
- I want to run a marathon and need to drop fifteen pounds to do so
- I have saved for two years and am going on a beach holiday and I want to look and feel great in my bikini
- I want to encourage my husband to eat and live in a healthier manner so that when he retires next year we can enjoy our time together

COMMANDMENTS

4. Getting 'attitude'

Going into a diet with the right attitude is key. Convincing yourself that you are signing on to weeks of suffering is a recipe for failure. So tell yourself you are going to have fun. Plan to embrace the new experience and consider any moments of weakness simply as challenges to be overcome. Arm yourself with the knowledge that THE NO CRAVE DIET is designed to make your weight-loss programme easier by reducing feelings of hunger and eliminating the overwhelming desire to snack that plagues most diets. Learn to enjoy your successes such as not giving in to a craving, feeling healthier and more energetic, and of course seeing your weight go down on the scales.

5. Writing a journal

For those of you who already write a journal of some kind, the value of such an exercise might readily be apparent. For those who do not, the concept of writing down your thoughts may seem a little bizarre, its purpose somewhat obscure. However, once you start, the simplicity of the process and its immediate and lasting value will rapidly be realised.

You have already had some practice writing your thoughts when you established your 'diet commandments'. For your journal the best way to start is when you feel a food craving start to edge its way into your day. Simply jot down what you are craving and how you are feeling at that moment. Think back over the past hour or so, the events leading up to the food craving. Try to express how you are feeling and understand what is driving you towards that unhealthy snack. Are you feeling overworked or overwhelmed, frustrated or angry, upset or depressed about something? Consider if you are really hungry or just snacking because you are bored! Continue your thoughts on paper, imagining how you will feel after the snack and later in the day. The likelihood is you will feel bad, not just because of the poor nutritional content of the snack but because you have cheated on your diet and broken your commitment to yourself.

And to make matters worse, the original cause of the craving has not been addressed! Recognising your craving patterns and the reasons behind them is the most important purpose of the journal. By examining how you feel, you reinforce the fact that eating a snack will not take away the emotion. In fact, you will end up feeling worse afterwards, both physically and mentally. Awareness and knowledge as to why you are craving a food is one of your best forms of defence to help combat the food munchies.

Once your journal is under way you can revisit different pages to learn your patterns of food craving. Go back and reread sections you think may be relevant when known emotions or familiar situations arise.

Use your journal for positive affirmation as well! Describe how you feel at the end of the first week when you step on the scales and find you have already lost a couple of pounds. Write down your successes at work, at home, emotionally or physically. Explain how you dealt with an issue, how you felt afterwards and what you would do differently next time. The journal can be as simple or as complex as you wish. Just make sure it balances the good with the bad, the easy with the difficult. And reread it often!

Julie's journal – an example

Wednesday:

Craving: I am craving a bag of chips. I am making dinner, fish and fresh vegetables, but right now I really want chips! Why?

My Day: Had a long day at work. Project deadline fast approaching and Jane is not pulling her weight. It feels as if the whole project rests on my shoulders. It took 1½ hours to get home because of an accident on the motorway and I skipped the gym.

Emotions: Tired, overwhelmed. I am hungry but dinner will be ready in 15 minutes. I need a snack because it is part of my 'letting down' process. I come home, I feel safe, I unwind and part of that always involves a snack.

How I change: Put on a CD of my favourite music. Sit for 10 minutes, relax, take some deep breaths and have a glass of water. I recognise that the project will be completed on time and that both John and Ellen have worked just as hard and have supported me throughout. Time for dinner.

6. Distract yourself

As we said before, most food cravings dissipate in ten minutes, so distracting your mind for a short time will allow the craving to pass harmlessly. Using your mind with a crossword or Sudoku, or reading a few pages of your current book is ideal. Or occupy your hands with knitting. Painting your nails is helpful as by the time they are dry and you can start snacking, the craving is long gone! Some people like to use movement to distract them, simply by getting up away from their desk and walking around the office, or moving away from the kitchen (and shut the doors to the kitchen) to remove the visual stimulus. Remember that most cravings are the brain's way of tricking you into eating food that it really doesn't need. Take control of your brain, give it something else to think about, and in doing so, you have now fooled your brain while winning the food-crave battle.

7. Teaming up with a buddy

When in doubt – get support from a friend. Everything in life is easier with the support of friends. Whether or not they are following **THE NO CRAVE DIET** with you, let your friends know what you are doing. Ask them for support so that when you go out in social situations, they help you stick to the programme, rather than encouraging you to deviate and share in the cake and crisps. In fact, it will benefit them too, for they may make better food choices in your presence as well.

Ask a friend to be your support buddy. A support buddy is someone you can call, email or talk to in person when you start to crave. Explain to them the No-Crave principles. They can help you rationalise why you really do not need that biscuit, and that by eating it, you will end up fighting more and more food cravings over the next few days. Having the support of someone there to tell you 'No' will reinforce your commitment, and his or her congratulations on your success will act as a reward. Not only will you have successfully beaten the craving, and prevented further cravings down the road, but you will also feel a sense of pride from both yourself and your buddy.

Ideally, you should choose a buddy who is also following **THE NO CRAVE DIET** because talking someone else out of a cheat helps to remind yourself of why you should not do it either. Mutual support and understanding of one another, recognition of your own and others' strengths and weaknesses is greatly beneficial when trying to see through your own food cravings and make the right choice.

Always carry the phone number or email address of your buddy so that no matter where you are or what you are doing, if you need their support, they can help you through.

8. Reward yourself

Like it or not, we all need rewards. The secret of success in your diet is to make those rewards calorie-free! When life is already stressful, a diet can often provide an unwanted extra challenge, something your reward centres feed on. So when you start **THE NO CRAVE DIET**, think of something that brings you pleasure. This may be a massage, a pedicure, coffee with a girlfriend or shopping. Try to work these rewards into your schedule.

Choose some that are routine, like meeting up with a friend once a week. Schedule that activity as you would any other appointment so you know that you always have time for it. Visiting a friend can be just the relief you need at the end of a day or week to relax, let your hair down, laugh and balance a hectic stressful life.

Then choose a reward that you would not normally do for yourself. This may be a new outfit you want, or a day at the spa. Then have a reward jar placed in your kitchen, or on your desk at work – somewhere you will see it during times of food cravings. Every time you beat that craving and don't give into it, place a pound or two inside that jar. Similarly, at the end of each successful day (whether or not you had a food craving is irrelevant), if you did not cheat, another pound or two goes in the jar. However, if you do cheat on any given day, or give in to a food craving, a pound must come out. At the end of a specific time frame that you have chosen (it could be at the end of each week, or each month) take the money out and treat yourself to something special. Seeing that jar fill up will encourage you to keep going. Watching it go down will be a reminder that you need to get back on track, or review the supplement and lifestyle sections of the book for extra support against food cravings.

9. Get enough sleep

You probably consider sleep the least useful part of your weight-loss programme. However, for a number of reasons, getting sufficient sleep is vital.

Reasons why sleep helps you lose weight:

■ Lack of sleep increases your hunger messenger (NPY)

■ Sleep deprivation increases the stress hormone cortisol, which makes you hungry

■ Lack of sleep lowers growth hormone, which promotes weight gain

■ Lack of sleep leads to more fat storage

■ You burn fat while you sleep

Sleep deprivation does not just refer to months of medical-student-style scheduling! A decrease of only one hour a night can have a detrimental effect on us. As part of **THE NO CRAVE DIET**, adequate sleep is essential. The number of hours' sleep each person needs is variable, but the majority of us need seven to nine hours.

Lack of adequate sleep has been shown to increase levels of the major hunger messenger (NPY) in the brain. This promotes food cravings and the desire to snack. Individuals working nights or needing to stay up late often snack. They are not sure why they feel hungry all night when normally they would be in bed, asleep, not even thinking about food. Sleep normally shuts down the hunger centre, allowing you to get adequate rest without waking up every hour to forage in the fridge.

There is a direct relationship between stress and impaired sleep patterns. To compound this effect, decreased sleep hours or decreased quality of sleep both lead to an increase in our stress hormone, cortisol, and this increase further disrupts our sleep pattern, creating a vicious cycle. The increased levels of cortisol make us feel hungrier all day. There is also a strong relationship between sleep deprivation and reduced levels of a growth hormone associated with weight gain and an impaired ability to burn fat. And of course, poor sleep means reduced energy, decreased immunity, weakness, impaired endurance, poor libido and high cholesterol.

The hormonal changes associated with insufficient sleep all contribute to altered metabolism with greater storage of sugar as fat and an impaired ability to break down our fat stores and use them as fuel. In addition, we know that night-time is actually a prime fat-burning time for the body. Once the calories from your evening meal have been used up you begin to burn your energy stores. Sleep really is an important part of your weight-loss regimen! Although you switch to fat-burning mode after three to four hours, there is a significant increase in this metabolism after about eight to nine hours following your evening meal. It stops the moment you eat breakfast. So, eating early allows your food to digest and promotes more restful sleep. It also gives you eleven to twelve hours before breakfast, which means three or four hours of prime night-time fat burning.

Here are some ways to make sure you get sufficient sleep:

- Reduce your stress levels: Reducing stress levels with deep breathing or meditation can be very useful. Bodywork such as massage therapy on a regular basis is also valuable at decreasing overall stress and promoting restful sleep. Aromatherapy can be used before bed. Burn a lavender candle or put a little lavender oil on your pillow. Supplements to help you sleep include melatonin, passionflower and hops (the herbal extract, not the beer).

- Get into a routine: Our body loves routine. Providing it with a rehearsed setting for sleep to take place is a valuable step towards a good night's sleep. This means getting into bed at about the same time each night.

- Dim the lights: Once we fall asleep our body starts to produce melatonin, our sleeping hormone. It changes our brain waves from the active beta waves to the calm theta waves of deep sleep. Production of this hormone is also linked to light and darkness. Our body will increase the production of melatonin when it is dark and suppress its production in the light. So try to make your room as dark as possible to mimic night-time and increase production of your sleeping hormone.

It is also wise not to spend your last hour before getting into bed under bright lights. This will hinder the secretion of melatonin and make sleep more difficult.

- Exercise: Try to avoid vigorous exercise in the evening, as this is likely to increase cortisol and other stimulatory hormones, which will make relaxation difficult.

- Food and drink: Eating early (between 5 p.m. and 6 p.m. if you plan to go to bed around 10 p.m.) will allow your food to digest before sleep and maximise the fat-burning time between dinner and breakfast. Avoid a large meal late in the evening, as it is likely to give you a higher than normal peak in glucose levels due to the inactivity that follows as you wind down for the evening. This will increase your hunger hormones, making you want to snack again before bed. Alcohol is also known to increase hunger hormones, so avoid this if you are having trouble sleeping. Caffeine in tea, coffee or soda can have a long-lasting stimulant effect, interfering with restful sleep. Try to avoid them after lunchtime and certainly during the evening.

10. Sex

Foods high in sugar and fat cause the brain to release more of the 'reward' messenger, dopamine. This makes you feel good, at least temporarily, and it is the rise in the dopamine these foods produce that attract us to them. For similar reasons, some individuals are attracted to smoking, gambling or shopping, as these activities can also increase dopamine. However, from the No-Crave point of view, there is one activity that increases your dopamine, makes you feel good, reduces hunger and helps you lose weight. Sex!

Of course, no one is recommending that you get amorous every time you feel the need to eat a cream cake or a bag of crisps! That might raise a few eyebrows on the bus! But within a caring, safe, healthy relationship, maintaining a healthy sex life can certainly help your diet. Sex, with or without orgasm, results in a peak in dopamine levels that will satisfy your reward centre, keeping your mind off of other satisfying treats like pudding! It will also decrease levels of your hunger hormone NPY, further reducing cravings. And you will be burning off calories!

10 emergency No-Crave measures

In the early stages of **THE NO CRAVE DIET**, your brain will still be used to feeling hungry, snacking between meals and getting regular rewards. It may take a few days for the diet to start eliminating these feelings, and that can make the first seven to ten days a little tough. There are plenty of 'Temptation Therapies' (see p.103) for you to try as well as some 'emergency' supplements (see p.131).

Food cravings can be beaten. Think of these as emergency measures. You will need them less and less as you progress with the diet and your cravings subside.

I have found that my patients employ many of these techniques in their day-to-day lives. Circumstances may dictate which are appropriate, but having different options means there is always a way to beat the cravings!

Increase your protein

By increasing the ratio of protein to carbohydrate in your diet, blood-sugar levels are stabilised, reducing the 'lows' that stimulate food cravings. In addition, a higher protein diet tends to promote a more acidic environment within the body, which in itself tends to reduce food cravings. If you really have to have something to snack on, have a small amount of protein. Five to ten grams is the equivalent of a third of most protein bars, or two tablespoons of cottage cheese. Unlike snacks high in sugar, starch or fat, protein will not induce further cravings and, as an added bonus, protein can increase your overall metabolic rate so you burn more calories!

Write them down

Simply jot down your craving and how you are feeling in a journal. Try to express how you are feeling and rationalise what is driving you towards that unhealthy snack. Evaluate what you have eaten so far today and plan your next meal. Continue your thoughts on paper, imagining how you will feel if you do have the snack and what it will mean later in the day. Remember that when you snacked in the past it made you feel unhealthy, relieved your hunger for only a very short period of time and encouraged you to repeat the snack again and again. Recognising your craving patterns and the reasons behind them is key.

Eat some fibre

Inulin or flax are zero glycaemic index fibres that stabilise blood-sugar levels and increase feelings of fullness without adding extra calories. Thus your stomach's stretch receptors will tell your brain you are full earlier and for longer, reducing hunger and cravings. It has other benefits such as stabilising bacterial flora in the bowel, improving motility and softening your stool. (For this reason, if you are prone to loose bowel movements this supplement should be avoided.) One teaspoon of inulin or defatted flax fibre in a glass of water is usually enough. Limit yourself, however, to one or two teaspoons per day.

Take a breath

Cravings are often the result of stress. A simple stress-relieving exercise is to sit back and take three to six long, slow breaths. It takes a little practice but once mastered your stress level can be instantly ameliorated. Close your eyes (if safe to do so!). Take five deep breaths. On your first inhalation, slowly count to three. Then start to exhale on a count of three. On the next breath, again inhale to three, and exhale to five. On the third and subsequent breaths, inhale to a count of three, and exhale to seven. (If you feel that you can comfortably increase the counts on either inhalation or exhalation, do so.)

Get moving

Most food cravings will dissipate within ten minutes of their onset. This is particularly true if you can get your endorphins and happy-hormone levels up. Exercise is ideal for this and does not have to involve a swift change into gym clothes and ten laps around the office! Simply getting up from your desk and walking around, stepping outside for a moment, or even working on some core exercises in your chair (see the Exercise section) will help take your mind off the food craving, and stop the physical desire (chemical messengers) that are leading you towards the doughnut box.

Drink some water

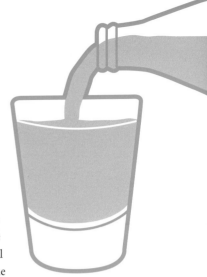

Cravings for food, and even feelings of hunger, are often caused by dehydration, so take a drink of water, herbal tea, decaffeinated coffee or your favourite low-calorie beverage. You will also stimulate stretch receptors in your stomach that will then send a message of satisfaction to the brain and stop the craving. Having a bottle or jug of water available at all times is key. Adding a few slices of citrus or cucumber to create a slight taste will enhance its effect, and in the case of grapefruit may actually directly inhibit cravings.

Phone a friend

Being on a diet is always easier with two! Calling a friend to tell them about your craving is half the battle towards overcoming it. Knowing that someone else is feeling the same way, along with hearing their words of encouragement, is a very valuable weapon in your armoury against cravings! I call it 'the buddy system'.

Read one of your diet commandments

At the beginning of your diet I encourage you to make a list of reasons why you want to lose weight. This list of 'commandments' may include everything from looking good in a swimsuit on holiday, to increasing your energy levels and reducing your blood pressure. Having your commandments handy and reading one or two at times of craving is very motivating.

Check your treat jar

Your treat jar is part of your diet incentive plan! Food cravings are all about reward, so rewarding yourself in ways that do not involve food is an easy way to reduce snacking. Adding a few pounds to the jar for each day you adhere to your diet allows you to save for a special treat at the end of the week, perhaps a new item of clothing or a massage. Giving in to a craving means taking money out, making that big reward harder to achieve.

L-glutamine

When you are hit with a food craving, particularly a sweet one, this simple amino acid can help eradicate it within thirty seconds. When we see a food that we desire, or think about a food we may wish to eat, our salivary glands begin to release digestive juices that interact with our taste buds, and send a message to our brain to further stimulate the urge to eat this food. L-glutamine interacts with the same taste receptors on the tongue to extinguish that message to the brain within seconds. If you feel unable to resist the biscuit or brownie you desire, open up a 500mg capsule of l-glutamine and put it directly on the tongue with a sip of water. Hold it in the mouth for about thirty seconds, and then swallow. You will be surprised how quickly the craving subsides. L-glutamine is also great for muscle and bowel repair, so you will also be doing your body a favour! You can easily take up to 5000mg a day if you need to, but remember, the longer you go without a specific type of food treat, the less you will desire it.

But if you really are at the end of your tether try one of the following

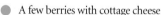

- A bite-sized square of protein bar – cut up a whole bar and keep the pieces wrapped separately so you are not tempted to have the whole bar
- A few vegetable sticks, with or without some dip
- A few nuts (about ten) – walnuts are best
- A couple of tablespoons of low-fat cottage or ricotta cheese
- A few berries with cottage cheese

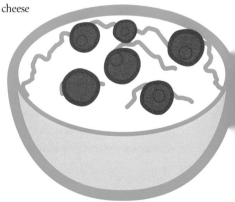

What to do if you cheat in Phase 1

- ■ Recognise your cheat
- ■ Remove the temptation
- ■ Eat some protein
- ■ Drink some water
- ■ Journal
- ■ Quick exercise
- ■ L-glutamine
- ■ Breathe in
- ■ Get back on track

No one is perfect. Even with the best intentions and the strongest desire to stay on track, life will undoubtedly present you with a situation that, despite your best efforts, you are unable to handle. It may be dinner at a friend's house where they have baked your favourite cake, or an unexpected glass of wine after work with a colleague that came with a bowl of crisps. Or it may be an unavoidable emotional event, which pushes all thoughts of a diet to the furthest recesses of your mind.

All my patients cheat once in a while. So, instead of feeling bad, know you are not the first and take a few simple steps to ameliorate the effects of that unhealthy snack and to decrease the risk of it happening again.

Recognise that it is only one cheat and stop right there. No one has ever failed a diet from just one cheat. Most people fail because they can't stop cheating. There is this underlying thought that one cheat ruins the whole day, so people will continue to cheat, and in fact gorge on food the whole day with the thought that tomorrow is a new day and they will restart fresh tomorrow. Drop that thought. Understand that there will be times when you fall off your diet plan, and just get right back on it.

Remove the temptation – if the source of the cheat remains close by, resisting another cheat will be more difficult. Put the biscuits or crisps away in a hard-to-reach cupboard or, better still, throw them out!

Protein – try to eat some protein as quickly as possible. Protein will slow down the delivery of sugar from your snack into the bloodstream and therefore decrease the excess release of insulin and subsequent weight gain. It will also help to prevent the hypoglycaemia (low blood sugar) that follows a sugar load, something that stresses the body and causes further food cravings. In addition, protein will change the pH levels in your mouth, altering the communication between your taste buds and your brain that would normally keep you coming back to the kitchen looking for more treats all night long.

You don't need a whole meal of protein to achieve this. Five to ten grams of protein, the equivalent of a third of most protein bars, or two tablespoons of cottage cheese will do the trick. Keep some handy!

Water – even if you do cheat, you will most likely not feel full. Cravings, after all, are about taste and reward, not about nutrition. The fact that you still feel hungry often leads to more snacking or even a full meal in order to satisfy that new sensation. Drinking water immediately after your cheat tricks the stretch receptors in your stomach into sending a message of satiation and satisfaction back up to the brain. This will stop your snacking before it gets out of control! Remember that citrus-infused water tastes and works better.

Journal – write down what you have just eaten so that later on you can clearly recognise the cheat. Then write down how you were feeling just before you ate the treat, both physically and emotionally. Most likely you were feeling thin, with a flat stomach, but stressed or fatigued. Then write down how you feel emotionally and physically after the cheat. Most likely you are still stressed and fatigued, but you now can add bloated, swollen and/or fat to the list! You can clearly see that you do not feel better – no one is ever satisfied after a cheat, and in fact you have just made the situation worse. Even though those few calories have not made any significant impact on your weight, you will feel as if they have.

Unless you clearly see these thoughts written down, you may not recognise the impact the cheat has had on you. Under normal circumstances we go right back to our busy schedule and ignore the unwell feeling in our body, only to feel worse and worse throughout the day. In addition, later on in the day, we usually attribute this worsened emotional and physical state to the stresses of our day rather than realising the impact that cheat has had on our body. By keeping a journal we can start to see patterns and prepare for them.

Exercise – if circumstances allow, try to do five minutes of exercise. A brisk walk is ideal. It will take your mind off further snacking and improve your mood.

L-glutamine – interacts with taste receptors on the tongue to extinguish the 'eat more' message to the brain within seconds. Open up a 500mg capsule of l-glutamine and put it directly on the tongue with a sip of water. Hold it in the mouth for about thirty seconds, and then swallow. This will reduce the size of your cheat and stop you going back for more.

Breathe – whilst cravings are often caused by stress, giving in to them can actually increase your stress afterwards. Recognise this and sit back to take a few deep breaths, realising that this one cheat is nothing to be upset about and knowing there are plenty of ways to stop it happening again. A simple stress-relieving exercise is to sit back and take three to six long, slow breaths. It takes a little practice but, once mastered, your stress level can be instantly improved. Close your eyes (if safe to do so). Take five deep breaths. On your first inhalation, slowly count to three. Then start to exhale on a count of three. On the next breath, again inhale to three, and exhale to five. On the third and subsequent breaths, inhale to a count of three, and exhale to seven. (If you feel you can comfortably increase the counts on either inhalation or exhalation, do so.)

Get back on track – do not dwell on your cheat. Move on and get back on track with your diet. Beating yourself up will just prolong the bad effects of the cheat by making you feel guilty or depressed, key triggers for more craving. Be positive and do not let the cheat get the better of you – become stronger in the knowledge that both **THE NO CRAVE DIET** and the numerous tips and lifestyle changes will inevitably make cravings and cheats a thing of the past. Most importantly, get back on track right away. Do not write off the rest of the day and fall completely off your diet by promising yourself you will start again tomorrow. Start right now!

Monitoring your progress
The rate of weight loss

The rate of weight loss, as with any change in the body, will vary between people. On average you will lose about two pounds per week. During the first week this may double or triple, with half of that loss being attributed to water. It is quite common to see larger losses one week followed by a smaller loss in the second. Some individuals even see large losses of four to five pounds a week for two or three weeks, followed by maybe a two-week plateau period without significant loss and then a return to a loss of four to five pounds per week. This cycle is repeated with rapid loss over a few weeks and then a short period of weight stability. If you are in this category, do not be discouraged by the plateau period. Be assured that by sticking to THE **NO CRAVE** DIET your weight loss will resume.

This is very safe and manageable level of weight loss. If it were any faster it would begin to drain your body of energy and place stress on other areas such as the immune system and the adrenal glands (stress glands). If it were any slower, it would be frustrating.

Healthy weight-loss guide – how long do I stay in Phase 1?

My patients lose an average of 18 to 22 pounds over 8 weeks in Phase 1 of THE **NO CRAVE** DIET.

1. If you are slightly overweight (ten to twelve pounds), I would recommend four to six weeks in Phase 1 with adjustment depending on your starting weight and rate of loss.

2. If you are fifteen pounds or more above your ideal weight, then you probably need the full eight weeks in Phase 1.

For those individuals wishing to lose more weight at the end of the eight-week period, simply continue with Phase 1 of the diet. The good news is that after the first six to eight weeks, cheating or straying temporarily from the diet will have much less impact on your weight loss. This is because, once you have retrained your metabolism, as long as you combine a cheat with protein (your body's new cue not to secrete excess insulin), you will no longer react hormonally to this food in the same way. Instead of storing this 'cheat' food as fat, you remain in a balanced blood-sugar state, and while you may not lose weight at that sitting, you do not have to worry about gaining!

Weekly weight and craving chart

To help you keep track of your weight, weigh yourself once a week. It is important not to weigh yourself every day. Very few people lose weight consistently each day, as there are fluctuations in your weight from water retention, salty food, hormones and the natural weight-loss process.

Over the course of a week, weight will increase and decrease slightly, but by the end of the week there should be, on average, a two-pound loss. This chart will allow you to monitor your weight loss.

In the chart below, write down the date you begin Phase 1 of THE NO CRAVE DIET. Next, record your starting weight. During the initial eight weeks of Phase 1 of the diet, try to weigh yourself on the same scales and at approximately the same time of day each week. This will help to ensure a more accurate weight reading. Monitor your craving level daily using a 1 to 5 scale, with 1 being no cravings and 5 representing unbearable cravings to which you may have given in.

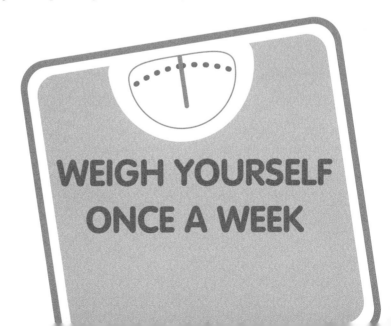

WEIGH YOURSELF ONCE A WEEK

THE **NO CRAVE** DIET

Starting date	/ /					Starting weight	
Craving Level	1	2	3	4	5		
Day 1							
Day 2							
Day 3							
Day 4							
Day 5							
Day 6							
Day 7							

Week 2 date	/ /					Week 2 weight	
Craving Level	1	2	3	4	5		
Day 1							
Day 2							
Day 3							
Day 4							
Day 5							
Day 6							
Day 7							

Week 3 date	/ /					Week 3 weight	
Craving Level	1	2	3	4	5		
Day 1							
Day 2							
Day 3							
Day 4							
Day 5							
Day 6							
Day 7							

Week 4 date ___/___/___   **Week 4 weight** _____

Craving Level	1	2	3	4	5
Day 1					
Day 2					
Day 3					
Day 4					
Day 5					
Day 6					
Day 7					

Week 5 date ___/___/___   **Week 5 weight** _____

Craving Level	1	2	3	4	5
Day 1					
Day 2					
Day 3					
Day 4					
Day 5					
Day 6					
Day 7					

Week 6 date ___/___/___   **Week 6 weight** _____

Craving Level	1	2	3	4	5
Day 1					
Day 2					
Day 3					
Day 4					
Day 5					
Day 6					
Day 7					

Week 7 date   /   /   **Week 7 weight**

Craving Level   1   2   3   4   5

Day 1

Day 2

Day 3

Day 4

Day 5

Day 6

Day 7

Week 8 date   /   /   **Week 8 weight**

Craving Level   1   2   3   4   5

Day 1

Day 2

Day 3

Day 4

Day 5

Day 6

Day 7

Supplements to minimise food cravings
What are natural supplements?

A few natural supplements can provide an optional addition to the fundamental dietary changes of the No-Crave plan. They can help reduce cravings, particularly during the early phase of the diet or during times of increased stress. They can assist blood-sugar control and fat burning. In my practice they provide an important part of my management plan for weight loss and reducing food cravings. You do not have to use them but I find that most of my patients like to know about them just in case. The supplements I recommend here take effect within three to four days, if not sooner.

Supplement quality

Supplement quality can vary substantially between manufacturers. We suggest using a reputable company specialising in health products. For more general information on supplements see the Resource section (see p.202).

When should I take them?

Generally I recommend taking supplements on an empty stomach for maximum absorption. Avoid taking them first thing in the morning; the best times are 10 a.m. and 2 p.m. (between meals). There are a few exceptions:

- Calcium–magnesium and CLA can be taken with food
- B-vitamins must be taken with food
- Melatonin should be taken before bed

What supplements should I start with?

Not everyone needs every supplement. I usually tailor an individual supplement plan for each patient depending on their specific weight loss and the types of food they crave.

However, I know from experience there are certain supplements that most people starting a diet and battling food cravings will find helpful. These five supplements can be taken safely to help decrease food cravings, encourage feelings of satisfaction, increase fat burning without stimulation and help retrain your metabolism into a fat-burning machine. None of these five have any adverse side effects. You will only do your body good while decreasing food cravings and increasing fat burning with these important nutrients.

- Green tea extract: 300mg twice a day
- Calcium–magnesium: 500mg of each twice a day
- Malic acid: 500mg twice a day
- L-carnosine: 500mg twice a day
- Multi B-vitamin: 100mg once a day

See the Supplement section for more details about these.

How long should I take them for?

In most cases I recommend taking any new supplement for a month (unless you notice side effects). However, if you find, for example, that your sweet craving has subsided after a couple of days, or your workplace stress has resolved, then try stopping them sooner and restart on an 'as needed' basis.

Supplements that reduce specific food cravings

Different supplements can be used for different cravings.

- Sweets: Increase your l-glutamine (open the 500mg capsule on your tongue) particularly around meal times and add 5-HTP 50–100mg twice a day (see caution in Supplement section for 5-HTP if you take any prescription medications).
- Fatty/savoury foods: Add in tyrosine 500–1000mg per day or CLA 500–1000 mg twice a day.
- General: Hoodia 400–800mg twice a day between meals and 5-HTP 50–100mg twice a day (see caution) can be used for general cravings.

Supplements that reduce your appetite

Although **THE NO CRAVE DIET** and basic supplements are highly effective at reducing your overall levels of hunger, some people do need a little extra help, especially in the early stages, around your period and when you are stressed. The following are excellent ways to reduce hunger pangs if they become a problem.

- Hoodia: 400–800mg twice a day between meals
- Inulin fibre: 1tsp–1tbsp twice a day
- L-carnosine: 500mg twice a day

Supplements that help stabilise blood sugar

If you find you are feeling hungry between meals, have low energy or are a little light-headed, you may need help stabilising your blood-sugar levels between meals. Until you get used to the protein message and correct your excess insulin, the level of glucose in your blood may get a little low between meals, particularly in the early stages of **THE NO CRAVE DIET**. Low blood sugar can also bring on food cravings so it is important to get this under control. I find the following supplements very useful.

- Chromium: 200 micrograms a day
- Melatonin: 3mg at night
- Inulin: 1tsp–1tbsp twice a day

Supplement Safety

Supplements, although natural, can have side effects and interactions with other medications (both natural and pharmaceutical). So check the label and, if you are concerned, discuss with your doctor, particularly if you are already on medication. Always inform any doctor or surgeon who treats you about every medication you are taking, natural or otherwise.

Supplements to reduce stress

Stress contributes to food cravings. Even the most ardent No-Crave dieter can be derailed by a stressful event at home or work. Your brain is tuned to reward and at times of stress, not only does the stress hormone cortisol encourage you to eat, your reward centre desires a perk to make up for the hardship. Being stressed can be one of the toughest times to encounter cravings. However, a combination of supplements and some of the simple lifestyle stress-managing exercises (see page 154) can minimise its impact on your diet.

- 5-HTP: 50–100mg twice a day
- Magnolia bark extract: 500mg twice a day
- Green tea extract: 300mg twice a day

Other supplements:

- GABA: 500mg twice a day
- Holy basil: 200mg twice a day
- Passion Flower: 500mg twice a day

Supplements for when you feel down

A depressed mood initiates food cravings, particularly for chocolate or sweets. Whether it is due to a severe bout of the flu, PMS, a work disappointment or relationship disaster, the feeling is the same. All you want to do is curl up in bed with a box of chocolates or a tub of ice cream. Try these supplements in your hour of need.

- 5-HTP: 50–100mg twice a day
- B-vitamins: Increase to 100mg twice a day
- Milk peptides: Increase your daily dose to 100–200mg twice a day or just take an extra 50mg when you feel sad
- Magnolia extract: 500mg twice a day

Chapter 4: Phase 2

The second phase of THE NO CRAVE DIET is the maintenance phase, a true lifestyle change that can be easily maintained for the rest of your life. Think of it as a healthy, enjoyable diet without the risk of regaining lost weight and battling food cravings!

During this phase you get to gradually reintroduce the restricted foods you gave up in Phase 1. Throughout this second phase, you will forget you ever had food cravings; your energy levels will remain high and your weight stable. You can enjoy every food group and continue to protect yourself against diet-related diseases at the same time. These benefits will last forever as long as you balance your protein and newly introduced carbohydrates at each meal. The maintenance phase is thus not so much a phase as it is a permanent healthy lifestyle change.

Reintroducing carbohydrates

During Phase 2 you can begin to reintroduce some of the carbohydrates that were eliminated or markedly reduced in the first phase. Now your body has consolidated the No-Crave message, it is possible to add in carbohydrates at a higher concentration, along with the protein, without increasing food cravings or weight. Because you have corrected your hormone and metabolic balance and have tamed the messengers in your brain that promote cravings, these foods will no longer be your enemy.

Note: It is not absolutely necessary to bring these restricted carbohydrates back into your diet on a daily basis. You may wish to have them only occasionally or not at all. It is your choice.

The order in which you reintroduce the carbohydrates is very important. You must slowly integrate them back into your diet in a particular pattern, and the sequence of reintroduction is determined by the sugar load found in each carbohydrate. Fructose, the sugar found in fruit, is the first to be introduced.

This is followed by glucose from whole grains and breads, then pasta, rice, potatoes and squash, and finally sweets and alcohol. Every two to three days you can move on to the next carbohydrate on the list. Adherence to this pattern minimises large jumps in blood-sugar levels and allows for easy adaptation of the body to carbohydrates.

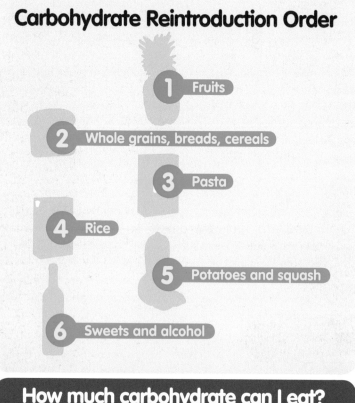

Carbohydrate Reintroduction Order

1 Fruits

2 Whole grains, breads, cereals

3 Pasta

4 Rice

5 Potatoes and squash

6 Sweets and alcohol

How much carbohydrate can I eat?

Unlimited Salads and vegetables	Phase I	Unlimited
	Phase II	Unlimited
Limited Vegetables and Legumes	Phase I	2 tablespoons every other day
	Phase II	Maximum 1:1 ratio with protein
Fruits	Phase I	2 pieces per day
	Phase II	Maximum 1:1 ratio with protein

Carbohydrate Chart
Carbohydrates reintroduced in Phase 2

Starches	Amount you eat to get 10 grams of carbohydrate	Amount you eat to get 30 grams of carbohydrate
Parsnips	1/2 cup	1 1/2 cups
Pumpkin	3/4 cup	2 1/4 cups
Rutabaga	3/4 cup	2 1/4 cups
Squash	1 cup	3 cups
Sweet Potato (baked)	3/4 cup	2 1/4 cups
White Potato (baked)	1/6 cup	1/2 cup
Chips (French fries)	5 fries	15 fries
Yam (baked)	1/4 cup	3/4 cup
Banana	1/3 banana	1 banana

Grains	Amount you eat to get 10 grams of carbohydrate	Amount you eat to get 30 grams of carbohydrate
Bagel	1/3 bagel	1 whole
Bread	1/2 slice	1 1/2 slices
Bun (hamburger or hotdog)	1/2 bun	1 1/2 buns
Couscous	1/4 cup	3/4 cup
Crackers (saltines/ Melba)	4 crackers	12 crackers
Tea Cake	1/3 cake	1 cake
Oatmeal	1/4 cup	3/4 cup
Pancakes	1/2 medium sized pancake	1 1/2 pancakes
Pizza (9 inch)	1/12 of the pizza	1/4 of the pizza
Rice (brown)	1/4 cup	3/4 cup
Rice (white)	1/4 cup	3/4 cup
Tortilla shell	1 shell	3 shells
Waffle (7 inch)	1/4 waffle	1/2 waffle

About the Phase 2 Carbohydrate Chart

The carbohydrate chart shows foods in the different carbohydrate categories and the amount of pure carbohydrate they contain. Please note that this chart is not intended to promote the weighing of food; that is not what THE **NO CRAVE** DIET is about. Rather, it allows you to make sensible choices about the foods you eat to better eliminate hunger and craving. Stay within your Phase-1 and Phase-2 food guidelines and choose foods in each category that allow you to eat a greater quantity while minimising carbohydrate intake.

For example, with reference to the carbohydrate chart on pages 42-43, in Phase 1 you can see that the unlimited carbohydrates (salads and vegetables) are 'unlimited' for a reason. You can have large amounts of them without consuming much carbohydrate – feel full without harming your metabolism. In Phase 1 you are allowed two fruits per day and a limited amount of higher-carbohydrate legumes. By referencing that table you can choose foods in this category that provide more volume for less carbohydrate. It is better to have a cup of blueberries or a whole peach rather than half an apple; they all have ten grams of carbohydrate but you get to eat more with the blueberries or the peach. Similarly, beets are a better option than chickpeas.

In Phase 2, when you reintroduce starches and grains to your meals, refer to the Phase 2 carbohydrate chart to make better food choices. For example, one cup of squash is more filling than half a slice of bread. You can also choose fruit over starch or grains, with nine apricots being equivalent to only fifteen chips.

How much carbohydrate?

The amount of carbohydrate you bring back into the diet is also very important. The total size of all the carbohydrate at one meal cannot be larger than the protein portion. As each new type of carbohydrate is reintroduced, you can increase the carbohydrate portion size until it is equal to your protein portion but no larger. A one-to-one ratio of protein to carbohydrate becomes your Phase-2 maximum. As you move down the list of reintroduced carbohydrates, they can be combined at one meal but the total combined carbohydrate portion must still not exceed the portion size of protein.

For example, suppose your protein portion size equals one hand-sized chicken breast:

- Days 1–3: add 1 extra piece of fruit (you are allowed 2 per day in Phase 1)

- Days 4–6: add a piece of toast (or half a slice of toast plus half an apple)

- Days 7–9: add half a cup of pasta (or a quarter-cup of pasta plus a slice of baguette)

- Days 10–12: add half a cup of rice (or a quarter-cup of rice plus half an apple)

- Days 13–15: add 2 small potatoes (or 1 potato plus a quarter-cup of rice)

- Days 16–19: add a glass of wine

Key things to remember for Phase 2

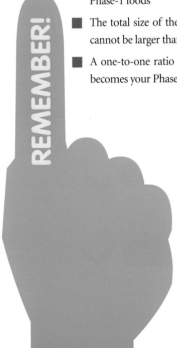

- You can continue with your unlimited salads and vegetables and other Phase-1 foods

- The total size of the previously restricted carbohydrate at one meal cannot be larger than the protein portion

- A one-to-one ratio of protein to previously restricted carbohydrate becomes your Phase-2 maximum

REMEMBER!

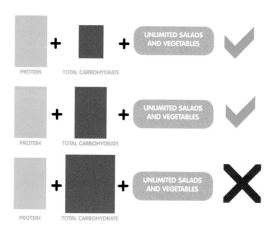

Your carbohydrate portion can contain different types of carbohydrate, but the total combined carbohydrate portion must still not exceed the portion size of protein.

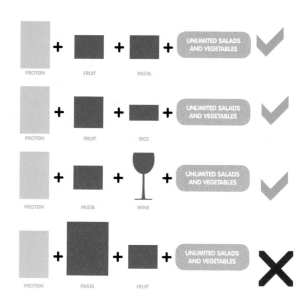

Signs that you are having too much carbohydrate

Your body will let you know if you ingest too much carbohydrate. Listening to these signs will prevent you slipping back into the type of diet that caused your metabolic and hormonal imbalance and overwhelming food cravings in the first place.

These signs are:

- Bloating after a meal
- Profound fatigue after a meal
- A return of feelings of hunger and cravings an hour or two after a meal
- Headache
- Dizziness or light-headedness

If these symptoms occur simply cut back your carbohydrate portion size and make sure you are maintaining adequate protein size.

Finding your Phase 2 balance

By following the Phase 2 guidelines above you will learn what your body's natural protein–carbohydrate balance should be. Everyone is a little different and some individuals will be able to tolerate more carbohydrate than others. Everyone, however, will be able to enjoy a varied and palatable menu including bread, pasta, potatoes, sweets and cake. As long as these carbohydrates are balanced with protein according to your Phase 2 balance you will not risk undoing all the good you did in Phase 1 or regaining all the weight you lost. However, once in Phase 2, don't be surprised if you fail to find all those carbohydrates appealing! Because you have your hunger and craving under control, your brain will adopt a 'take it or leave it' attitude towards those starchy, fatty foods you once held so dear. And if you don't miss them, don't eat them. They are not particularly nutritious and leaving them off your plate of grilled chicken and fresh salad will leave room for an extra glass of wine!

No-Crave Diet Phase 2 Summary

1. **Continue at one gram of protein per kilogram of body weight per meal**

2. **Continue unlimited salad/vegetables**

3. **Reintroduce restricted carbohydrates, with the following conditions:**

   - **Type:** Follow the order listed above

   - **Amount:** Increase slowly to a maximum portion equal to that of your protein at each meal

   - **Adjust:** Watch for symptoms indicating that you are having too much carbohydrate and not enough protein

How to keep the weight off and still enjoy your food

One of the greatest benefits of **THE NO CRAVE DIET** is the ability to enjoy a healthy, varied diet for the rest of your life without the fear that the weight you lost during Phase 1 will return. Most diets, and in particular the ones that rely on severe calorie deprivation, do not retrain your metabolism, so as soon as you stop and begin a more normal diet, the weight returns. Considering that these diets are the ones that produce the most hunger and craving, the rapid return of any lost weight is most depressing given the suffering you have endured. With **THE NO CRAVE DIET**, the metabolic retraining in Phase 1 means you can begin to enjoy a more varied menu in Phase 2 without that worry. In addition, the eradication of cravings means you will feel much more in control of what you eat, so less likely to settle back into old habits. Of course we are not pretending that once in Phase 2 you can do anything you like! There are still some basic rules and a diet consisting of fast food, processed meals, excess carbohydrate and too much fat will eventually shift your metabolism back to its unhealthy state and the weight will creep back. However, Phase 2 does allow great flexibility in your daily diet along with occasional wild nights of Bacchanalian delight!

Moments of weakness in Phase 2

There are two excellent pieces of news at this point. Firstly, by the time you reach Phase 2 the anti-craving effects of **THE NO CRAVE DIET** will be firmly established, meaning hunger pangs and food cravings will no longer be part of your life. Secondly, once in Phase 2, your ability to withstand a particularly wild night out is greatly improved. You are free to enjoy yourself without feeling guilty or worrying about reversing all the good you did early on. Even an entire meal of carbohydrates washed down with a few glasses of wine will not 'undo' the metabolic and hormonal retraining you have achieved. Any weight gained will be mostly water and is rapidly lost over the next few days on your regular Phase-2 maintenance menu. You won't even crave the next day – in fact quite the opposite! A note of caution, however. Continuing to eat in this way for three weeks or more will eventually undo the metabolic message your body has learned, and this will lead to weight gain and a return of food cravings. To reverse this effect you would then need to spend the equivalent number of weeks back in Phase 1 of **THE NO CRAVE DIET**.

Chapter 5: The No-Crave Exercise and Anti-Stress Plan

When do I start?

The first and probably most important message is that while exercise and stress management are important, you should certainly have Phase 1 and possibly Phase 2 comfortably under your belt before embarking on this part. What we are saying is, do not try to do everything at once. Concentrate on THE NO CRAVE DIET: it is the most important aspect of your new lifestyle. Attempting to change your diet, start a new exercise regimen and incorporate stress-management techniques into your life all at the same time is overwhelming and likely to reduce your ability to stick with any one programme. What is more reasonable during Phases 1 and 2 is to add in some of the more simple suggestions from this section, for example taking the stairs rather than the lift or getting a massage once every couple of weeks. That way you get some of the benefits of exercise and stress management without trying to organise a complete schedule.

The second message is also important. Exercise and stress reduction will help you lose weight, reduce hunger and food cravings, and improve your health. So they are a valuable part of your No-Crave programme. So introduce them, but only when you are ready. That may be a few weeks into Phase 1 or later in Phase 2. Just fit them into your schedule once you feel you have the diet under control.

The No-Crave benefits of exercise

First, the good news! The most important factor in THE NO CRAVE DIET is what you eat and when you eat. In fact, 70 to 85 per cent of your daily calories are used up by simply being and staying alive –sitting, lying in the bath, sleeping – by changing what and when you eat THE NO CRAVE DIET corrects imbalances in your metabolism that will make you store less fat and burn more fat.

And now the better news! Exercise can enhance THE NO CRAVE DIET not only by burning extra calories but also by staving off cravings. For those of you who have never exercised, or only exercise occasionally, there is no need to be alarmed. We are not insisting on a two-hour boot camp every day! The No-Crave Exercise Plan incorporates simple ways to exercise and increase your heart rate starting with only twenty minutes three times a week.

The benefits of exercise include:

- Reduces appetite and craving
- Stimulates the same reward messengers as a sweet snack
- Improves your mood and attitude
- Builds muscle that burns more fat
- Increases your metabolism
- Increases the number of calories you burn
- Improves cardiovascular health
- Maintains strong bones

Increasing your metabolism and calories burned

Any physical exercise will increase your metabolism both during the activity and for a short time afterwards. Following thirty minutes of regular exercise your metabolic rate can take up to one hour to return to normal. So you get ninety minutes of calorie burning for only thirty minutes exercise – that's like finding a fabulous deal in the January sales! The amount by which you increase your metabolism depends on the type of exercise you do. Obviously the more vigorous the activity the greater the increase in metabolism, but any exercise will offer the same benefits to your diet, your weight and your health. So start slowly and work up – you'll be surprised how quickly you begin to increase your fitness and how soon your exercise programme will become as normal a part of your day as brushing your teeth.

30' exercise = 90' burning calories

The No-Crave Exercise Plan does incorporate specific exercises, but reference to the chart below will show you that some activities you tend to do on a regular basis about the home or at work count as exercise and can be substituted for step-ups, walking or jogging.

Activity	Calories burned in 20 minutes (77kg/12st individual)	% increase in calories burned over resting
Resting/Sitting	40	0
Walking	100	250
Tai Chi	100	250
Gardening	100	250
Vacuuming	94	235
Carpentry	94	235
Fishing	81	203
Hatha Yoga	67	167
Tennis	189	473

Exercise reduces appetite and craving

You may have already tried the 'Get moving' option in '10 emergency No-Crave measures', so you know how effective even a brief period of activity is at turning off your hunger centre. The reasons are simple. Exercise increases activity in areas of the brain associated with 'fight or flight', your sympathetic pathways. From an evolutionary perspective they are much more concerned with you evading a potential threat than getting your hands on a double-cheeseburger. So the hunger centre is turned off and your cravings subside. Of course there is no real threat (except perhaps to your waistline), but the brain is tricked into shutting down your desire to eat. Regular daily exercise will have the same effect, and the longer and more vigorous the activity, the more profound and long-lasting the suppression of your hunger centre.

Your brain sees exercise as a reward

Besides turning off your hunger centre, exercise has a number of other effects on messengers in the brain. One of the most important is the stimulation of your reward centre through increased production of our happy, feel-good hormones, dopamine and serotonin, along with our natural opiates, the enkephalins. This effect is the same as that induced by sugary or fatty snacks and treats, and is part of the reward system in the brain. So, by providing your brain with the reward chemicals it craves through exercise rather than unhealthy snacks you continue to feel good, eliminate craving for food, lose weight and improve your health.

Exercise makes you feel good

Believe it or not, exercise is actually going to make you feel good. Besides knowing that you are increasing your metabolism, burning calories and reducing your cravings, exercise causes your brain to release 'happy hormones'. Dopamine, serotonin and the enkephalins all contribute to a sense of wellbeing, enhanced mood and positive attitude. They make you feel in control, in charge of your body, no longer at the mercy of food cravings and the need to overeat.

More muscle burns more fat

The cells in your body need energy and therefore burn calories all day every day whatever you are doing, even resting or sleeping. That is why 60 to 75 per cent of the calories we burn each day come from simply being alive. (The figure of 70 to 85 per cent given at the start of this section includes an extra 5 to 10 per cent burned eating, digesting and storing the food we eat.) This resting metabolic rate is dependent upon a number of factors including your age, sex and body composition. The more muscle you have, the higher your resting metabolic rate and the more calories you burn at rest.

Cells burn calories at different rates. Fat cells, for example, burn calories at only a fraction the rate of a muscle cell. A pound of fat might use up only 1 to 3 calories per day, whereas a pound of muscle will burn up to 120 calories a day. The reason is that muscle cells have a far higher content of the body's powerhouse components, the mitochondria, millions of tiny energy-combusting units in every cell.

All exercise uses muscle activity and to a certain extent will increase muscle mass. However, certain exercises, particularly core strength and weights training, will actually increase your muscle mass significantly, allowing you to burn more calories even at rest. Of course we are not talking about turning you into the next Mr or Ms Universe, simply replacing some excess soft spots with useful firm muscle.

Heart health and strong bones

Exercise has been shown to lower cholesterol and reduces your risk of cardiovascular disease, type-2 diabetes, high blood pressure and stroke. It has also been shown to reduce your risk of developing certain types of cancer (colon, prostate, uterus and breast). In addition it helps prevent depression, back pain and osteoporosis (thinning of the bones). Exercise reduces stress and helps you sleep better. All in all, besides its benefits to your diet, it seems like a generally good idea!

Simple ways to increase exercise

There are some simple ways to exercise without starting a formal workout regimen. They are useful when you are just starting **THE NO CRAVE DIET** and do not want to juggle too many new things at the same time.

- Walk to work if it is a reasonable distance
- If you take a bus or train walk to a stop that is a little further away before getting on or get off a stop earlier
- Take the stairs rather than the lift or escalator
- Go for a walk at lunchtime rather than sitting in the cafeteria
- Walk to get the paper in the morning
- Wash your car by hand once a week

Exercise Hints

- Do exercise you enjoy – you are more likely to stick with it
- Exercise with a friend for added motivation
- Use music or a video as distraction
- Set aside a specific time for your exercise rather than trying to fit it in 'when you get a spare moment'

Your own home exercise routine

Note: Before you start any new exercise programme we recommend you check with your family doctor.

If you already exercise regularly then this section might be of interest simply to add a few new exercises or routines to your week. If you have never or only rarely exercised then the No-Crave Exercise Plan offers you an easy way to incorporate activity into your life. For the many reasons mentioned above, exercise will enhance THE NO CRAVE DIET, producing faster results and an even healthier you. It will always be easy to make excuses as to why you didn't exercise; what you need to do is find reasons you should. Try making a list of some of the benefits above, those you feel are most relevant to you, and read them just before you decide to skip your routine for the day.

If you are not used to exercising, getting into a routine can be tough. For that reason we start you off with a schedule that can easily fit into your week: twenty to thirty minutes, three times a week. This is a minimum, and it provides a starting point for you to work with. We know your lifestyle is hectic and you have to balance home, work and family, so this allows you to incorporate exercise with minimal disruption. That way you are more likely to start! Eventually we would like to see you doing some type of exercise for thirty to forty minutes, five times a week, inclusive of aerobic activity and weight training, but for now let us start with something simple.

During the beginning stages of exercise, it is important to focus more on cardio than strength training exercises. It is also crucial that you work out at your own pace. Each exercise listed below can be adapted to increase or decrease the intensity according to your fitness level. As you gain more strength and endurance, you can increase both the time spent exercising as well as the intensity. First begin with at least twenty minutes three times a week. Make at least one of the days an alternating circuit of cardio and strength training. The other two days can be cardio alone, or more circuits with different exercises. Below is an example of a twenty-minute cardio/strength training circuit. Not only can you vary the types of exercises in the circuit (see ideas in the lists below) but you can also vary the intensity of each exercise. For example, push-ups can be done on the ground either from your toes, on your knees, or standing up and leaning against the wall. On-the-spot walking can be done at a slow or fast pace, and bringing your knees up higher will make it more energetic.

Before and after your workout

If you plan to do a twenty- to thirty-minute workout make sure you set aside time for your exercise. Wear loose, comfortable clothing and cushioned, supportive shoes. The more you 'psych' yourself up for exercise the more likely you are to enjoy it and put more effort in. Exercise science tells us that even during the preparation phase of exercise (getting dressed, thinking about your drill), your heart rate and metabolism will increase – and incidentally any hunger or food craving will subside. This is one of the reasons why exercise is a good 'Temptation Therapy'.

Putting on some of your favourite music or watching a TV show while working out will make the exercise seem to go faster, as your mind is distracted. Have a watch or clock easily visible so you can monitor your progress.

Start with a slow-paced exercise to warm up, and do more cardio than weights or strength training when you first begin to exercise. As you progress, you can add in more weight training, or even hire a personal trainer to help tailor a workout specific to you and your needs.

At the end of your workout do some deep breathing and use some of the simple stretches illustrated below.

Simple Home Workout

Start by alternating exercises from the lists below. To begin, choose one cardio exercise for two minutes as a warm-up. Then switch to an upper-body strength exercise for thirty seconds, then back to a cardio exercise for one minute followed by lower-body exercise for thirty seconds, back to a cardio exercise for one minute and finally an abdominal exercise for thirty seconds. Then repeat the cycle until you have completed a minimum of fifteen minutes. Use the last five minutes for a two-minute cardio warm-down followed by stretching.

So your twenty-minute routine should be:

4' cardio exercise warm-up

30" upper-body exercise

1' cardio exercise

30" lower-body exercise

1' cardio exercise

30" abdominal/core exercise

1' cardio exercise

30" upper-body exercise

1' cardio exercise

30" lower-body exercise

1' cardio exercise

30" abdominal/core exercise

1' cardio exercise

30" upper-body exercise

1' cardio exercise

30" lower-body exercise

1' cardio exercise

30" abdominal/core exercise

4' cardio warm-down

Stretching

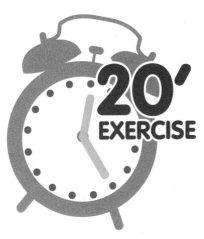

Sample Exercises

These exercises are designed to be performed anywhere. You do not need a gym or special equipment.

The table below shows exercises in each of the four categories:

- Cardio exercise
- Upper-body exercise
- Lower-body exercise
- Abdominal/core exercise

Within each category are three levels of exercise: easy, medium and hard. During your workout you can choose any exercise from a category and select the difficulty level. As you get fitter you can progress to the more difficult exercises.

Alternative cardio exercise

On some days you may wish to intersperse other forms of exercise as an alternative to your home circuit. Examples include:

- A twenty-minute walk at a speed that increases your heart rate
- Cycling for twenty minutes
- Gardening for thirty minutes
- Cleaning the house, including vacuuming, for thirty minutes
- Dancing for twenty minutes
- Swimming for twenty minutes

Exercise	Easy	Medium	Hard
Cardio			
Walking on the spot	Slow walk	Fast walk	Bring knees to chest
Step to the side	Legs only	Legs plus arms	Star jumps
Knee lifts	Knee to waist	Knee to chest	Knee to chest plus arms
Step ups	Step forward on flat	Step up small step	Step up large steps
Forward kick	Low kick	High kick	High kick plus arms
Upper body			
Push-ups	Against a wall (standing)	Knees on the ground	Regular (toes on the ground)
Biceps	No weight	Can of soup in each hand	5 pound weight
Lateral raise (to just below shoulder height)	No weight	Can of soup in each hand	5 pound weight
Shoulder press	No weight	Can of soup in each hand	5 pound weight
Triceps	No weight	Can of soup in each hand	5 pound weight
Lower body			
Standing Squat	Knees bend to 45 degrees	Knees bend to 90 degrees	Knees to 90 degrees with weight
Lunges	Step forward short distance	Step forward long distance	Step forward long distance with weight
Side leg lifts	Up and down	Hold for 2 seconds	Hold for 5 seconds
Sitting leg raise	Up and down	Hold for 2 seconds	Hold for 5 seconds
Abdominal/Core Exercises			
Lying on the floor, knees bent	Tilt pelvis, contract abs	Lift shoulders from ground	Lift shoulder and hold 2 seconds
Lying on floor, legs supported	Tilt pelvis, contract abs	Lift shoulders from ground	Elbows to knees crunch
Abdominal Plank	Up and down	Hold for 2 seconds	Hold for 5 seconds
On all-fours	Lift 1 arm or 1 leg	Lift 1 arm or 1 leg and hold 2 seconds	Lift 1 arm and opposite leg
Lying on stomach	Lift 1 arm or 1 leg	Lift 1 arm and opposite leg	Lift both arms and both legs

The No-Crave anti-stress plan

Chronic Stress is not 'normal'

Stress has become such an overused word in our society that it is now considered normal. In fact, it is considered almost abnormal if we are not stressed. We may even feel guilty if we are relaxing, or not being productive in some way. We have learned to equate productivity and success with being busy, and being busy with increased stress. Therefore, in order to be successful, we must be stressed. However, in association with this success, we live an unhealthy lifestyle including poor diet and lack of exercise, the combination forming what is often termed 'overindulgence syndrome'. Chronic stress causes metabolic changes that lead to weight gain. Over the long term, this abnormal state can lead to the complex of symptoms termed 'metabolic syndrome', including obesity, diabetes, high blood pressure and cardiovascular disease.

The body's response to stress is necessary for our survival. We are designed to react quickly to stressful situations, either to fend off or flee from danger. This is called the 'fight or flight' response. This specific reaction takes place every single time our body senses stress of any kind. It doesn't matter whether the stressful situation is real or perceived, physical or psychological, once our brain interprets a situation as stressful the reaction is the same. The glands responsible for producing stress hormones cannot differentiate between the stress of a wedding or a funeral. They will react in a similar manner to a physical threat, increased workload at the office, financial difficulty, or a relationship problem. Whatever the stressor may be, the final reaction is the same, the fight-or-flight response.

Caveman vs. Downtown Man

You are probably familiar with the scenario typically used to teach the principles of stress. A prehistoric 'caveman' meanders along, minding his own business, wondering whether to wear the bison or the bearskin loincloth for dinner, when a sabre-toothed tiger leaps out of the bushes. The fight-or-flight mechanism is activated. Adrenaline kicks in, causing the caveman's pupils to dilate, his heart and breathing rate to jump, skin to go cold, and the hair to stand up. Muscles twitch in anticipation of the next move. Senses are heightened.

The caveman throws a rock (fight), then jumps quickly into a gully (flight), running as fast as he can, powered by the surge of energy from increased levels of blood sugar. By now, cortisol, the major stress hormone, is beginning to rise, supporting the initial adrenaline rush to permit a prolonged reaction to the inherent danger. Cortisol is more potent and long-lasting than adrenaline, with profound effects at the cellular level.

In just moments, the threat is over. The tiger has stopped pursuing the man, distracted by a passing rabbit, which proves to be a more accessible prey. With a sigh of relief, the danger past and his cave in sight, the caveman's alarm system turns off. The stress hormones stabilise his body before switching off and returning to normal levels. The mechanism has worked, enabling survival in the face of danger and restoring his life to normal with no ill effects apart from a battered prehistoric ego!

Now, several thousands of years later, 'downtown man', tired from a sleepless night, has already battled with what he perceives as the first stressful situation of the day – whether to wear the Armani or Prada power suit to the corporate merger presentation – and is now sitting in traffic, fifteen minutes late for work. His mobile phone rings. It's his boss, informing him that if he's late, he might as well not show up at all. No one to fight, nowhere to flee. Reaching to put the phone down, he knocks his coffee over the presentation sheets on the passenger seat. The traffic hasn't moved an inch. Despite the fact that none of this is anywhere near as dangerous as confronting a sabre-toothed tiger, he perceives it as a threat, his brain programmed to interpret such situations as 'stressful'.

Unfortunately for downtown man, the primitive areas of the brain and their associated hormonal reactions have not progressed much since his loincloth days. Once the fight-or-flight mechanism kicks into action the cascade of adrenaline and cortisol begins, raising heart rate, blood pressure and breathing. Unfortunately, unlike the first scenario, downtown man's stressful situation does not resolve quickly and when it does, another one rapidly replaces it. This chronic stimulation of the stress response leads to increased hunger, food cravings and weight.

Stress promotes weight gain and food craving

Chronic stimulation of the stress reaction leads to hormonal and metabolic imbalances that adversely affect all systems in the body and lead to excessive weight gain. In particular chronic stress promotes weight gain around our mid-section, stomach, hips, buttocks and upper thighs. Besides being undesirable this specific fat distribution is most associated with serious health problems, including type-2 diabetes, high blood pressure and heart disease. In addition, stress interferes with our hunger and satiety messengers, causing an increase in food cravings. It makes us seek out 'comfort' foods high in sugar and fat to try and placate our jittery nervous system and then encourages our body to store the extra calories as fat around our tummies.

Stress:

- Stimulates the hunger centre
- Desestabilises blood sugar and increases cravings
- Makes us resistant to our anti-hunger messengers
- Increases levels of hunger hormones
- Reduces our 'happy hormone' levels, which increases craving

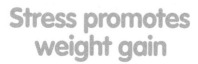

Stress promotes weight gain

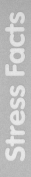

Stress Facts

Did You Know?

The Institute of Personnel and Development says sickness leave is costing British Industry £500 per employee – that's £13 billion a year. It claims 6.5 million sick days are being taken every year as a result of stress.

In a recent survey 89 per cent of respondents described experiencing 'high levels of stress'. Stress is very expensive. It is recognised as the No. 1 killer today.

Are You Stressed?

Some people seem to cope with stress better than others, for reasons that aren't always clear.

They seem to have a great gift for completely 'turning off' their mental thought processes when they get into bed, despite the very important business meeting they have at 9 a.m. the next morning. Other people are not as fortunate – or relaxed. How many times have you lain awake in bed at night trying desperately to fall asleep? The more you try, the harder it becomes. Then you start worrying about that meeting, exam or interview the next morning and how you must get some sleep to prepare for it.

The fact that you aren't sleeping then becomes yet another stressor and ultimately makes the entire situation worse. If you are lucky enough to fall asleep, you find yourself wide awake between 2 and 4 a.m. and begin the entire process all over again. You feel and hear your heart beat as you lie there in bed trying to count those sheep jumping over the fence. If any of these events sound familiar, read on.

Attitudes towards stress

Here is a sample of different attitudes towards stress, some healthier than others.

'I know I'm stressed most of the time'

You have already made it over the first hurdle. You are listening to your body and know you are stressed. You may already know some of the ill effects that stress causes. This book will both expand your knowledge of stress-related disease and allow you to reduce your own personal stress level.

'I'm occasionally stressed, but that's normal'

Being stressed once in a while is definitely part of life, but that does not necessarily mean it is healthy. Even brief, regular stressful episodes can have a detrimental effect on your wellbeing, and the likelihood is that many of these stressors remain unresolved, causing a low level of chronic, unrecognised stress.

'I don't think I'm stressed'

Of course, we realise there are individuals who remain 'cool, calm and collected' through all adversity and they may indeed have their stress response under control. Others may have lifestyles free from the rigours of modern-day life, have perfect family and personal relationships, and a happy work environment.

We suspect, however, that these individuals are the exception rather than the rule. Most people who believe they are not stressed have not taken a close look at their life and their health and are not listening to their body. They attribute their fatigue, recurrent colds, anxiety attacks and skin rashes to other factors, ignoring the hectic pace at which they live. Recognising the 'red flags' of chronic stress and learning how illness and stress are related is vital for this category of individual. Having realised that 'perhaps I am a little stressed', simple lifestyle changes can be instituted to enhance awareness of your body's response to stress, along with a plan to control it.

'I am stressed but I thrive on it'

Sound familiar? At the gym by 5 a.m. and in the office by 7 a.m. Lunch on the fly. Leave work at 8 p.m., head out for drinks and dinner. Party until 2 a.m., then head home for a couple of hours sleep before starting again. With catchphrases like, 'I work better under stress' and 'I only need four hours sleep a night', these individuals are invincible – or at least they think they are!

No doubt about it, when you're young, your body will put up with more or less anything you throw at it. However, while you seem to be able to cope with stress much better, the damage to your health is already being done. Take a look at your boss! Overweight, high blood pressure, diabetes, stomach ulcers? That could be you in ten years time. While we do not expect you to settle into a middle-aged lifestyle at 22, we hope to institute some simple changes that will keep you healthy so you can enjoy that time when it comes!

Stress Checklist

Many people suffer from chronic stress but do not realise it. It may be an important contributor to your weight gain and your difficulty losing pounds, and is certainly responsible for many of your unexplained food cravings.

If any of the following symptoms are familiar then you need to address your chronic stress issue as part of your personal No-Crave plan:

- Weight gain principally in the mid-section of your body
- Waking up tired in the morning despite seemingly adequate sleep hours
- Difficulty falling asleep, waking between 2 and 4 a.m., often restless with racing thoughts
- Frequent irritability with episodes of anger
- Anxiety attacks
- Constant worry or fear about life
- Jaw clenching or teeth grinding
- Frequent colds and flu

- Heart palpitations, high blood pressure and heart disease
- Slow recovery from illness or injury
- Bowel irritability or irregularity
- Frequent headaches or migraines
- Poor concentration and memory
- Feeling overwhelmed at work or at home
- Depression or episodes of despair or weepiness
- Irregular menstrual cycles
- Reduced libido
- Difficulty getting pregnant despite normal test results

How THE **NO CRAVE** DIET reduces stress

You may be wondering how starting on THE **NO CRAVE** DIET could possibly help reduce your stress levels. You may have tried other diets before and found that your stress levels actually increased. Worrying about calories, ounces of fat and carbohydrate indexes along with the trauma of persistent food cravings probably only exacerbated your daily stress. Fortunately, following THE **NO CRAVE** DIET will actually reduce the stress load on your body and, by combining it with some of the simple lifestyle techniques or supplements, you can look forward to a thinner, calmer you!

Reducing Stress on THE **NO CRAVE** DIET

THE **NO CRAVE** DIET reduces stress on the body by:

- Stabilising blood sugar levels
- Letting you use your food as fuel
- Correcting insulin and leptin resistance
- Reducing hunger and craving

It uses simple techniques to reduce stress:

- ◼ Exercise
- ◼ Deep-breathing exercises
- ◼ Meditation
- ◼ Yoga or Tai Chi
- ◼ Bodywork such as massage or aromatherapy

It can recommend supplements to reduce stress:

- ◼ Green tea extract
- ◼ Magnolia flower extract
- ◼ 5-HTP
- ◼ Passionflower
- ◼ Holy basil

THE **NO CRAVE** DIET actually reduces stress!

As mentioned before, it is hard to imagine that any type of diet could actually reduce the stress in your life. However, the metabolic effects of THE **NO CRAVE** DIET substantially reduce some of the major stressors on your brain and tissues, stressors you may not even be aware of. For example, the wide swings in blood sugar that occur with our poor diet and dysfunctional metabolism impose a stress on the body as significant as a confrontation with an aggressive animal. Yet because of the nature of this type of stressor (physiologic as opposed to physical) you will be unaware it is actually occurring. In a sense this is a much more dangerous type of stress, as without the awareness that it is occurring you are unlikely to do anything about it. Fortunately once you start THE **NO CRAVE** DIET your blood-sugar levels will automatically become more stable without the stressful highs and lows. This in itself produces a significant reduction in stress to the body.

Additional metabolic effects of THE **NO CRAVE** DIET also reduce physiologic stress on the body. Allowing you to use your food as fuel means there is a constant supply of energy for your brain and tissues, preventing fatigue and exhaustion. Correcting resistance to the hormones insulin and leptin allow your metabolism to function more efficiently, responding normally to the messages the body provides about food intake and energy supplies. Again, this will stabilise blood sugar, maximise your energy levels and prevent excess fat storage, which stresses organs, muscles and joints.

Finally, **THE NO CRAVE DIET** reduces your hunger and food cravings. This removes a significant stress from your life, allowing you to continue the diet without feeling as if every day is a battle with a sabre-toothed cream cake!

Pick and Mix techniques for reducing stress

Reducing the level of stress in your life does not have to be difficult. There are many simple lifestyle changes and exercises that can have a significant impact on both acute and chronic stress.

Instant Stress Relievers for acute stress

- Deep breaths – take five slow, deep breaths with your eyes shut (if practical). This is a quick version of the deep-breathing exercise below and will work best once you have practised the full exercise.

- Visualisation – write down the name of one of your 'relaxation places' and spend a few minutes visualising it. Further details are explained in the visualisation exercise below.

- 3-minute seated meditation (see below)

- Put on some of your favourite music, close your eyes and listen

- Play with your pet if you have one – studies show this to be an extremely effective stress reducer

- Take a quick walk – even simple exercise helps relieve stress

Daily techniques to relieve chronic stress

Exercise

Making exercise part of your daily routine is probably one of the simplest and most effective stress-reducing techniques. Whether a brisk walk, a swim, exercises in the home or a trip to the gym, all exercise helps decrease cortisol levels, promote a feeling of wellbeing and improve mood. In addition it has the added benefit of burning calories!

Yoga and Tai Chi are both forms of exercise and stress-relieving therapies, an ideal combination for the stressed No-Crave dieter.

Yoga

Yoga is best known as a physical practice utilising gentle stretching, breathing and relaxation techniques. Each of these techniques follows a specific pattern or sequence that helps to relax the mind and energise the body. Practice begins with concentration on breathing to quiet the mind. When the mind is quiet, the release of cortisol, our stress hormone, decreases. There next follows a series of gentle movements and poses that helps to strengthen and lengthen the muscles. This also helps to increase the circulation through the body, which in turn provides new nutrients to damaged or inflamed areas of the body and removes toxins.

There are essentially no contraindications for yoga. Some people may need to limit the range of motion through some of the exercises. Such caution is advised in the presence of a total hip replacement (due to decreased stability in the joint). This should be discussed with your surgeon. Some individuals may need to begin more slowly with the exercises and build up their strength and flexibility. It is important not to push the body too far. Pain on a movement is indicative that you should move through the exercise with care.

Tai Chi

Tai Chi is often referred to as a moving form of yoga combined with meditation. There are many different forms of Tai Chi, otherwise known as 'sets', each consisting of a different sequence of co-ordinated movements. These movements mimic the natural movements seen in animals and birds, but unlike the staccato movements of these animals, Tai Chi is performed in a slow, continuous, even motion. Many of the movements stem from various martial arts practices, such as Qi Gong. Tai Chi has been used therapeutically with the elderly and injured for decades and has spread to all ages as a form of 'warm-up', cross-training, and body-awareness exercise. According to Tai Chi practitioners, you can easily reach the American Health Association standards for exercise by practising Tai Chi three times a day.

Deep breathing

Deep breathing can quickly become part of your daily routine. You may wish to deep breathe for five minutes in the morning before you leave for work, when you get home or just before bed. In addition, the technique can be used during the day to alleviate stress and anxiety.

Deep-breathing steps

1. Find a quiet, comfortable place to sit. Turn off distractions such as radio, television or telephone. Rest your hands on your knees or clasp them lightly in your lap.

2. Close your eyes and let your mind be aware that it is time to relax. Repeating a word such as 'calm' or 'peace' a few times may help at this point.

3. Become aware of your breathing. Rather than it being an automatic activity occurring in the background, concentrate on each breath. Feel the air entering and leaving your lungs over four or five breaths.

4. Breathe in through your nose and out through your mouth to start with and then, as your breathing deepens and you start to relax, in and out through your nose.

5. Try to breathe more deeply, using your diaphragm and abdomen rather than just your lungs.

6. As your breaths get deeper, pause very briefly between inhaling and exhaling, being aware at that point of the oxygen and energy filling your body.

7. Then pause slightly between exhaling and inhaling, allowing your body to completely relax at that very moment.

8. Try counting during inhalation and exhalation. Start with a count of three on breathing in and five on breathing out. If this feels comfortable increase the exhalation count a little at first and then the inhalation count.

9. As you breathe feel yourself relaxing, sinking deeper into the chair.

10. Continue for as long as you wish.

11. On completion of the exercise, open your eyes, return your breathing towards normal, and stretch. Bring your arms out straight then raise them slowly above your head, allowing them to touch before bringing them back to your side. Do this three times.

12. Get up slowly and in stages.

Note: During the exercise, do not hyperventilate. If you begin to feel dizzy or sick, open your eyes and stop the exercise. Concentrate on something else until your breathing returns to normal and any untoward sensations have passed.

Visualisation

This is another technique used to help both your mind and body relax by providing it with positive thoughts and temporarily steering the thoughts away from the 'worries' of your world. It is believed your thoughts influence how you feel and act. If you continually dwell on the negative thoughts and processes, then you are more likely to be an unhappy and unsatisfied person. However, if you change those thoughts into happy and positive ones, your mood and behaviour will most likely follow that change. Visualisation is a therapy used to help elevate your mood and direct your thoughts to positive ones.

Visualisation exercise

1. Start by sitting quietly and thinking of a place or an object that is pleasing to you, for instance a waterfall. Then begin to visualise all of the surroundings. Imagine the water rushing down and falling into the pool below. Then look up to see the mountains surrounding the pool and follow the pool of water down a stream, picturing the flowers and the trees along the banks.

2. Next imagine how the air smells, the sounds you may hear, and how the soft grass feels beneath your feet as you walk alongside the river.

3. As you move along, you can hear yourself saying, 'I feel calm,' or 'I am letting go of my tension and see it float away down the river.'

4. Once your body learns to associate this place with a feeling of relaxation and happiness, you can go to this place anytime you feel nervous, anxious or depressed and replace those negative feelings with calm ones.

Meditation

Meditation comprises a number of practices that aim to calm and quiet the active mind. By concentrating on one particular element, such as a sound, an image, a word or one's breathing, intrusive thoughts liable to induce stress are excluded.

Most people fill their mind with constant thoughts of past memories or future plans. Both have a tremendous ability to induce stress and disturb calm. The objective of meditating is to focus the mind on the present, allowing the body to feel, breathe and exist in the 'here and now', rather than in the past or future.

During meditation, we are not trying to remove all external stimulation. However, while experiencing and appreciating sounds, smells and images, they are allowed to drift through the mind without being dwelt upon.

How to meditate

While there are many different meditation disciplines (Transcendental Meditation, Zen Buddhist, Kundalini Yoga, etc.), they all share a few essential principles and practices.

Quietness and Isolation: You need to be somewhere where you will not be disturbed by other people, or devices such as telephones, pagers, radio or television.

Comfort: You need to be comfortable in your posture, clothing and environment.

Time: You need to set aside a certain amount of time that you are comfortable with. Whether you choose three minutes or thirty minutes, you need to complete the entire time period.

Attitude: You need to be open to the process of meditation and its desired goals. Peace and happiness are an ideal starting point.

Breathing: A key component to all meditation exercises is calm and controlled breathing. This can be practised first.

Do not be disheartened if your first attempts at meditation seem to be a battle of wills between you and the thought processes of your active mind. This is very normal and will subside as you get more experienced. Recognise the intrusive thoughts for what they are and let them drift by like clouds in a blue summer sky without dwelling upon them.

Hint: meditation tapes or CDs are an excellent way to introduce yourself to this form of relaxation.

Three-minute seated meditation

Once practised, this meditation can be used almost anywhere, allowing you the ability to calm your mind and body throughout the day. You should first learn this technique at home in a comfortable quiet place, but later on it may be used at work or on a train, for example.

1. Find a room where you can sit comfortably. You may choose to sit in a chair to support your back, or you may prefer to sit cross-legged upon the floor.

2. Wear loose, comfortable clothing, but ensure you are not too warm or too cold.

3. Turn off the television, radio or other devices, and unplug the telephone.

4. You may play some music which natural sounds such as ocean waves or forest sounds.

5. Close your eyes.

6. Take five deep breaths. On your first inhalation, slowly count to three. Then start to exhale on a count of three. On the next breath, again inhale to three, and exhale to five. On the third and subsequent breaths, inhale to a count of three, and exhale to seven. (If you feel you can comfortably increase the counts on either inhalation or exhalation, do so.)

7. While continuing to breathe, now concentrate on relaxing muscle groups throughout your body. Start with your forehead and face. As you exhale, feel the muscles in this area calm and relax. Release all tension from them. This may take a few breaths to complete. Then move on to your shoulders and perform the same exercise. Gradually work your way down through your trunk, along your legs, and finally into your toes.

8. Once you are completely relaxed, continue to breathe and focus on your breath as it moves freely through the relaxed muscles. Remember to breathe deeply, using your diaphragm.

9. On completion of the exercise, open your eyes, slightly increase your breathing, and begin to slowly move your limbs before standing. Do not stand straight up; rather, do it in stages to allow your body to adapt.

Lifestyle changes to reduce your daily stress

Lifestyle changes do not mean leaving your job, your family and your home, disposing of your earthly possessions and sitting cross-legged at the top of a mountain somewhere. Not only is it impractical, it is also quite uncomfortable!

Instead, introduce a little more simplicity into your life, recognising what is most important and trying to establish priorities. You cannot do everything and be all things to all people. You owe it to yourself to make your health your priority.

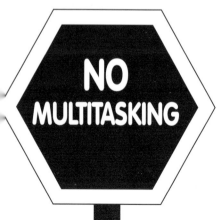

No multi-tasking

Do not multi-task. Although you may think this is a time-efficient way to go about things, you will rapidly become overloaded. The more stimuli you impose upon yourself, the greater the activity of your stress glands. Keep your tasks or jobs simple: that means one at a time, and do them well. When you are finished move on to the next.

Learn to say 'No'

People often have a problem saying no to others for fear of hurting or upsetting them. They end up saying yes to everything, taking on too much and hurting themselves. Learn what your boundaries are, and how much you can handle. Once you reach that limit, do not take on any more. Others will understand, for they themselves are on overload, otherwise they would not be asking for your help.

Avoid known stressors

If there are certain parts of your day where you know you will encounter stressors, try to alter your pattern. For instance, if you get upset in traffic try not to leave the house at rush hour. Get up a little earlier so you can miss the traffic – and possibly go for a workout before you start work. Then you can leave the office sooner and miss the traffic on the way home. If you can't avoid the traffic, then prepare yourself for it. Bring some soothing music to listen to, or a tape of something you want to learn. At least then if you are sitting in traffic, you can enjoy yourself.

Don't set unrealistic goals

Many of us want to do everything and do it as quickly as possible. We are impatient. Our society has programmed us to expect results straight away, whether that be in health care, a career advancement, or via high-speed Internet! Our failure to achieve goals is a major stressor. Reset your goals to be attainable, and attainable within realistic time frames.

Positive affirmation

Wake up and look in the mirror and take note of one positive thing a day. If you see something you don't like, then look away for now. Don't focus on the negative. Try to find something positive in everything, however hard that may seem. The actual process of looking for 'good' is calming – and finding it will improve your mood and outlook.

Bodywork

Physical therapies performed on you by a practitioner are termed 'bodywork' and include massage therapy, aromatherapy, reflexology, acupuncture, shiatsu and reiki. Their role in the management of chronic stress cannot be overstated. These techniques provide a direct and immediate reduction in stress along with numerous other benefits to the body. If possible they should become part of your new lower-stress lifestyle.

Massage

By reducing stress and increasing your feel-good brain hormones, dopamine and serotonin, massage makes you more relaxed, happier and less hungry.

Massage therapy is defined as the treatment of disease or injury through the manual manipulation of body tissues. Massage is employed for the relief of pain and spasm, to induce relaxation, to stretch and break down scarring and adhesions, and to increase circulation and metabolism. Massage promotes the resorption and metabolism of toxins and the residua of inflammation. The basic movements include effleurage, petrissage, friction, tapotement, and vibration.

Contraindications are few. Following acute injury or a severe flare-up of an existing injury, or in the presence of an open wound, local massage would not be advisable in that area. However, distant massage or massage therapy performed on other parts of the body is advisable to help increase the effects of the immune system and decrease inflammatory mediators, and cortisol levels. In order to receive these benefits, massage can be performed anywhere on the body. It is avoided in certain cancers to avoid promoting spread.

Aromatherapy

Aromatic healing oils can be used during a therapeutic massage. These essential oils are absorbed both through inhalation and through the skin during a treatment. Throughout the massage, lymphatic drainage, muscle releases and spinal pressures are applied to target the nervous system, and affect every organ and muscle of the body. Each oil has a different effect, ranging from detoxification and relaxation to increasing energy levels.

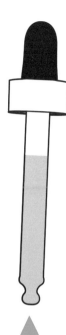

Essential aromatherapy oils for relaxation and stress relief are:

- Amber
- Bergamot
- Camphor
- Cedarwood
- Lavender
- Poppy
- Ylang-ylang

Essential oils can be used in various ways:

- Diffuser – a small metal bowl heated by a candle
- A few drops in a warm bath
- In a massage oil
- A few drops in a facecloth or sponge in the shower
- As a perfume

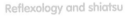

Reflexology and shiatsu

Reflexology involves the massage and application of pressure to specific area of the feet, while shiatsu employs the application of pressure to specific points throughout the body corresponding to specific acupuncture points along various energy meridians in the body. Both treatments are performed with you fully clothed and can be as short as ten minutes or as long as an hour. The relaxation effect is augmented by the release of 'reward' messengers, which further reduce hunger and craving.

Supplements to reduce stress

Certain supplements can be used safely to augment the stress-relieving effects of **THE NO CRAVE DIET**, your lifestyle changes and relaxation exercises. They are not essential but some individuals find them useful on a short-term basis to either kick-start their stress-reduction programme or to help during periods of increased stress in their lives.

Supplements to reduce stress are:

1. Green tea extract – 300mg twice a day
2. Magnolia bark extract – 500mg twice a day
3. 5-HTP – 50–100mg twice a day
4. Passionflower – 500mg twice a day
5. Holy basil – 200mg twice a day
6. GABA – 500mg twice a day

Green Tea

Buddhist monks originally brought green tea to Japan from China. It was quickly embraced by the Japanese as a soothing, calming drink and was rapidly found to have numerous health benefits. Today green tea is recognised all over the world for its therapeutic properties.

Green tea comes from the same plant as traditional black tea, *Camellia sinesis*, and is produced by steaming and drying fresh tea leaves at elevated temperatures in order to keep the active ingredients intact.

One of the active ingredients of green tea, catechin, boosts metabolism, increases calorie burning and promotes fat utilisation. Unlike other dietary stimulants like caffeine or ephedra, green tea increases metabolism without any increase in heart rate or blood pressure. Green tea extract also acts on certain receptors in the gut, reducing feelings of hunger and food cravings.

From a health viewpoint, green tea contains powerful antioxidants and has six times more antioxidant activity than regular black tea. Antioxidants help to decrease the cellular and DNA damage caused by environmental toxins that are thought to promote the progression of age-related illness such as cardiovascular disease, cancer and macular degeneration.

Dose: 300mg of green tea extract (standardised to 20 per cent of the active ingredient EGCG) twice a day on an empty stomach. Drinking green tea as an infusion is an alternative but is much weaker than the supplement form, the dose is hard to control and the added caffeine may cause side effects.

Safety: Very few side effects have been seen with green tea extracts or the tea itself. However, as they both contain caffeine, if you are highly sensitive to this ingredient, you may experience palpitations, increased sweating or anxiety similar to when drinking a cup of coffee. The tea leaves themselves contain far more caffeine than the supplement pills, so if you are concerned try the supplement before the tea itself. You can also try a decaffeinated version of the tea.

Magnolia bark extract

Magnolia bark is a traditional Chinese herb. In Chinese medicine it has been used since 100AD for treating what the Chinese refer to as blocked or stagnated qi (pronounced 'chee'). Qi in Chinese medicine is the energy and life force of the body. When qi is blocked it causes symptoms such as low energy, emotional distress or anxiety, digestive complaints, dizziness and alterations in the sleep cycle. In Western medicine this would equal stress and fatigue.

In both forms of medicine magnolia bark is used as a general anti-stress and anti-anxiety herb. Magnolia bark extracts do not have any sedating effects but most people do sleep more soundly when taking them.

Dose: For the average 140- to 150-pound adult, 500mg of extract twice a day on an empty stomach.

Safety: No side effects have been seen with magnolia bark extract. In some people who are used to high stress, fatigue may ensue for the first couple of days. It is important to note that this is not sedation, but rather a return to normal energy levels, not the falsely elevated energy levels we often refer to as an adrenaline high.

5-HTP

5-HTP, or 5-hydroxytryptophan, is one of the most important neurotransmitters in the brain. It is a close relative of serotonin, our happy hormone, and therefore aids in wellbeing, relaxation and stress relief. Chocolate and sweets make you feel good as they promote the release of serotonin and 5-HTP in the brain. This feel-good effect is what you crave. So by taking a natural supplement you cut out the cake-eating step and still get to feel good!

Low serotonin levels are associated with depressed mood, which explains why we crave sweets when life is not going so well. 5-HTP is a useful supplement at times like this as well as during times of stress when it exerts a calming effect, improving relaxation and sleep.

> Dose: For general relief of anxiety, 50 to 100mg twice a day is sufficient.
>
> Safety: Do not take if you are on prescription anti-depressant or anti-anxiety medication.

Passionflower

Passionflower (*Passiflora incarnata*) has been used medicinally for centuries, as a sedative by the Aztecs and as an antispasmodic and anxiolytic stress reliever by Europeans. Some of the first clinical studies were performed in Italy, where passionflower was observed to decrease brain excitation and prolong sleeping hours with no adverse side effects.

In France, a multi-centre study of anxious patients was carried out to evaluate a plant extract containing botanicals including passionflower. The plant extract produced significantly greater improvement in symptoms than the placebo.

> Dose: 500mg of dried herb twice a day. Passionflower is most frequently prescribed in combination with other herbs.

Holy basil

Holy basil or *Ocimum sanctum* is a herb native to India, where it is known as *tulsi*. Traditionally, holy basil is used for its anti-inflammatory properties in the treatment of asthma and respiratory illnesses. However, it has now been found to have significant anti-stress activity.

Holy basil is used extensively as an adaptogenic herb that supports and enhances the body's response to physical and emotional stress. It is used extensively as one of the primary botanical medicines in Ayurvedic medicine. Research demonstrates that holy basil safely lowers cortisol levels while regulating both the emotional and physical response to stress and supporting adrenal function at the same time. In addition holy basil helps maintain normal blood sugar and lower cholesterol levels and is therefore used clinically to help in the treatment of diabetes.

Dose: 200mg twice a day on an empty stomach.

See the Resources section for more information on these supplements.

Supplement Safety

Supplements, although natural, can have side effects and interactions with other medications (both natural and pharmaceutical). So check the label and, if you are concerned, discuss with your doctor, particularly if you are already on medication. Always inform any doctor or surgeon who treats you about every medication you are taking, natural or otherwise.

PART III

Resources and References

The science behind THE NO CRAVE DIET

This section is for those of you who want to discover a little bit more about why THE NO CRAVE DIET works. It answers questions such as:

- How can a diet actually reduce cravings?
- How can changing when you eat increases fat burning?
- Why is eliminating snacking important for weight loss?
- Why do certain foods actually increase hunger and craving?
- How do artificial sweeteners make me gain weight?
- What are the health benefits of THE NO CRAVE DIET?
- What has reward got to do with hunger and craving?
- What is the science behind hunger and satiety?
- What is the science behind stress and weight gain?
- Why do we crave a bacon sarnie after a heavy night out?
- Why does overdoing the bananas give you the munchies?
- What makes our bodies more likely to store fat than burn it off?

How THE NO CRAVE DIET reduces cravings

One of the most important ways in which THE NO CRAVE DIET reduces cravings is through stabilisation of blood sugar levels. Hypoglycaemia (low blood sugar) is a major factor in the development of food cravings. Stabilising blood sugar levels eliminates this disruptive influence on your diet. In the longer term, the diet reverses a metabolic abnormality widespread in our 21st-century society, a factor called insulin resistance. Insulin resistance makes your brain insensitive to the anti-hunger action of insulin. Reversing it through THE NO CRAVE DIET will return your metabolism to its normal, healthy state and allow the insulin released when you eat to adequately signal the brain to shut off your hunger and cravings.

Another factor responsible for hunger and cravings is resistance to the fat-messenger hormone leptin. Leptin is produced by fat cells once they are 'full' and should have a strong anti-hunger effect on the brain. This messenger is supposed to let us know when our energy stores are full and there is no longer a need to keep eating. Unfortunately, for a number of reasons, including our dietary habits, we have developed an insensitivity to leptin, resulting in hunger and cravings in the presence of more-than-adequate fat stores. Leptin plays a key role in stopping feelings of hunger late in the evening and overnight, and resistance results in the classic 'midnight munchies' trip to the fridge. Rebalancing your metabolism through THE **NO CRAVE** DIET, and reversing your resistance to leptin, will prevent cravings and snacking.

THE **NO CRAVE** DIET results in slower release of sugar into the blood and slower release of food from the stomach. You subsequently feel full longer and produce less of the potent hunger hormone ghrelin. Ghrelin is a messenger released by cells in the stomach once it is empty and is responsible for some of the hunger pangs and cravings between meals. Reducing the amount and period of time over which this hormone is released will make you less hungry and, subsequently, less prone to snacking.

Changing your metabolism means you can access your energy stores more easily. For example, hyperinsulinaemia (persistent high insulin levels resulting from a carbohydrate-heavy diet) prevents you breaking down your fat stores into high-energy value fatty acids, which can be used as fuel. Reversing this metabolic abnormality with THE **NO CRAVE** DIET improves your fat-burning potential and ability to lose weight. If you can access your energy stores easily, your body will not crave sugars between meals and you will actually burn off your fat!

How changing when you eat reduces craving and increases fat burning

THE **NO CRAVE** DIET works not only by changing what you eat but when you eat. The principal reason why snacking between meals promotes craving and impairs our ability to lose weight relates to our blood sugar levels and the hormone insulin. Once a meal starts, there is a rapid release of insulin over five to fifteen minutes, followed by a more sustained release for up to three hours. Once insulin is released, it promotes storage of food, especially sugar from the meal. This primitive design is aimed to make the most of any incoming food. Because food was scarce, storing it for future use was insurance against an unsuccessful hunt. Between meals, the liver should release its stores of glucose, keeping blood sugar levels constant. However, with constant snacking this mechanism is disrupted. Each meal, however small, causes insulin to be produced and, as a result, the pancreas, the gland that produces insulin, becomes exhausted. It can no longer provide the initial five to fifteen minute burst, instead producing a lower but more prolonged insulin release lasting beyond our original three-hour timeline. This lowers our blood sugar typically causing low energy, fatigue, hunger and craving about three to four hours after a meal. The liver, which should be producing sugar to maintain a more constant blood sugar level, is also not working properly. Because we keep artificially raising our blood sugar with snacks, it never gets the chance to make its own so it gets lazy and cannot deliver when asked. To add to our problems, it also gets angry and starts producing extra cholesterol!

Finally, snacking impairs the ability of our 'stop eating' anti-hunger hormone leptin to work. Leptin acts as a post-meal messenger to the brain, turning off our hunger for a few hours. This is most important at night. Eating frequent meals makes us insensitive to the effects of leptin so we ignore its message and continue to feel hungry between meals.

Reducing snacking improves fat burning

- Retraining your metabolism allows you to access your fat stores and use them for fuel
- Being able to avoid snacks between meals improves the fat burning that typically begins three hours after a meal
- Better sleep and no 'midnight munchies' allow you to access your night-time fat-burning potential

In order to lose weight we need to lose fat. Unfortunately, the only way to do this, besides under the care of your plastic surgeon, is to use it as an energy source. Your body's metabolism is actually designed to do this, but through poor diet and progressive weight gain you have turned off the pathways that metabolise fat stores. Retraining your metabolism, as mentioned before, goes a long way towards allowing your body to access these fat stores as a fuel source. However, there are other aspects of the diet that will further enhance this innate pathway.

As we noted, once we start to eat we release the storage hormone insulin.

Unfortunately, while insulin is working we cannot burn any of our excess fat as the hormone effectively blocks access to it. It is not until three hours later, once insulin levels have fallen, that we begin to be able to break down the fat on our hips and thighs and use it as fuel.

The problem with snacking between meals is that we never actually reach that 'three hour' mark. As soon as we start our snack, however small it may be, we start to pump out insulin. So instead of burning off our fat stores, we burn off the snack and save the hips and thighs for later. Of course 'later' never comes. In addition, when we keep asking the pancreas for more insulin it becomes depleted, eliminating that initial five to fifteen minute peak. The result is a lower but more prolonged insulin release taking us way beyond our original three-hour timeline. Eating just three good meals per day with 5 to 6 hours between them is a vital part of the No-Crave plan.

Night-time is actually a prime fat-burning time for the body. Once the calories from your evening meal have been used up you begin to burn your energy stores. You may think that just lying in bed sleeping is not exactly the most energetic part of the day. However, it is during sleep that the body regenerates and heals so your metabolism remains very active. And remember: your largest source of energy expenditure by far is your metabolism. It accounts for up to 85 per cent of the calories you burn each day, with the remaining 15 per cent a result of any exercise you do. Even a vigorous workout will likely only increase this to 20 per cent! So sleep really is an important part of your weightloss regimen. Although you switch to fat-burning mode after three to four hours, there is a significant increase in this metabolism after about eight to nine hours following your evening meal. It stops the moment you eat breakfast. So, eating early in the evening allows your food to digest and promotes more restful sleep It also gives you eleven to twelve hours before breakfast, which means three to four hours of prime night-time fat burning. The No-Crave plan allows you to achieve this without the late-night snack that would normally disrupt this valuable process.

Why certain foods increase hunger and craving

High fat and high sugar diets reduce the responsiveness of the brain to messengers that signal feelings of fullness. Normally these chemicals would cause a reduction in hunger and craving, but under the influence of fat and sugar, higher levels are required to exert the same feeling of fullness. The overall effect is to promote hunger and craving.

Diets that are high in saturated fats have been shown to promote activity in the 'hunger centre', increasing production and sensitivity to hunger and craving chemicals (NPY, AGRP and the orexins). This enhances our desire to eat and tendency to put on weight.

Diets high in saturated fats have been shown to act in two ways to increase hunger and promote snacking. They reduce levels of the signalling messenger (CCK) produced in the intestines during a meal, so you take longer to feel full. In addition they reduce the production and sensitivity of the brain to another chemical (α-MSH). This is probably the most important central messenger within the brain that inhibits the hunger centre and stops food cravings, so any reduction in its activity will have a profound effect on promoting cravings.

Thus a high fat, high sugar diet overrides our normal control mechanisms. By swinging the balance in favour of 'hunger' rather than 'satiety', meal size and duration is increased causing us to overeat and gain weight. Our 'balance point' is subsequently shifted to the left, making it even more difficult for us to swing it back to the right. Control of appetite and weight loss therefore becomes more difficult.

Increased hunger and Craving centre activity
Decreased satiety centre activity

Decreased hunger and Craving centre activity
Increased satiety centre activity

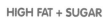

HIGH FAT + SUGAR

Feel Hungry
Crave and search for food
Eat
Save energy
Store fat

Not Hungry
Rest
Do not eat
Burn energy
Use fat stores

Summary

● High fat, high sugar diets induce insulin resistance, which impairs the ability of insulin to act as a satiety factor to reduce cravings.

● High fat diets lead to leptin resistance, which not only reduces its effect as an appetite suppressor, but also enhances our taste for sweet foods. (Leptin normally acts to inhibit the response to sweet taste.)

● Diets high in saturated fats increase production and response to hunger and craving-inducing chemicals.

● The response to 'I'm full' messengers is reduced by a high fat and sugar diet.

● A diet high in saturated fats reduces production and sensitivity to α-MSH, the most important anti-craving messenger.

In order to swing the balance back to the right we need to make changes to our diet. Besides being inherently healthier, it will allow our satiety mechanisms to function more effectively. Initially these changes need to be quite substantial: removing simple carbohydrates, sugars and as much saturated fat from our food as possible. This will allow our messengers to rebalance themselves and work more effectively, retraining them after years of improper function. Once achieved, we can carefully reintroduce some sugars and fats, but at a much lower level, otherwise we will once again disrupt our signalling system. Changing your diet to include less sugar and fat will automatically reduce your cravings as these foods actually promote snacking and the desire for more unhealthy foods.

Artificial sweeteners make you gain weight

You may think that using an artificial sweetener is a healthy option. However, in addition to the side effects of these chemicals, they are not going to help you lose your cravings. In fact, the evidence indicates that they may actually increase them.

There are two types of artificial sweeteners used as sugar substitutes in foods: non-caloric sweeteners and sugar alcohols. Non-caloric sweeteners include saccharine and aspartame. They do not add calories and are used widely in snack foods and drinks. Sugar alcohols include sorbitol and mannitol. They contain about the same number of calories as sugar, and are used in chewing gums, cough syrups, jams and hard sweets. Because sugar alcohols are absorbed and metabolised more slowly by the body than regular sugar, they were thought to be a viable sugar substitute for people with diabetes. However, it has now been shown that, once absorbed, they provide exactly the same number of calories as regular sugar. As such, sugar alcohols do not help people who are trying to lose weight.

Artificial sweeteners and weight gain

For those on **THE NO CRAVE DIET**, however, there is another reason not to consume these artificial sweeteners – they may actually make you gain weight! These so-called low-calorie or no-calorie sweeteners can disrupt the body's natural ability to judge the calorific content of a food by its sweetness.

In preparation for digestion and the hormonal response to food, the body asks, 'Will this food provide me with sufficient energy? Do I store this food as fat?' Taste buds on the tongue sense the sweetness of the incoming food and determine from there a rough estimate of the amount of sugar it will provide the body. Before artificial sweeteners were invented, sweet foods contained a large number of calories so the brain received a message telling it to turn off the hunger centre as very little of this food would be needed to restore energy. In addition it signalled to the pancreas to pump out more insulin to help deal with the incoming sugar load. The system worked because the sweetness of the food was a reliable and predictable measure of the number of calories that were about to be consumed.

Unfortunately, with the growing use of artificial sweeteners, our bodies have learned that they can no longer rely on sweetness as an accurate measurement of calories. Instead, the body has learned that very sweet foods do not actually contain as many calories as they should. Therefore, when we eat sweet foods, with real sugar or artificial non-caloric sweeteners, the brain no longer switches off the hunger centre quickly. It believes that, despite the apparent sweetness, we have not really consumed many calories and, therefore, continues to send out messages from the hunger and craving centres instructing you to eat more and more. Of course, the foods with artificial sweeteners actually contain lots of calories in the form of starch or fat, but the body is unable to sense these until much later. As a result, we consume far more calories than we should.

There are several studies confirming this. In one study, two groups of rats were given two differently sweetened fluids. The first group received fluid with a normal high-calorie sugar sweetener. The second group was fed fluid with non-caloric saccharin. After ten days the rats were allowed to eat a high calorie chocolate-flavoured food. The first group (regular sugar) ate limited amounts of the chocolate, sufficient for their caloric needs. The second group (artificial sweeteners), unable to interpret the caloric content of the chocolate, overate and put on weight.

What artificial sweetener should I look for?

There are really only two types of sweeteners that are low calorie and do not have a detrimental effect on the body. They are stevia and xylitol. These sweeteners, if placed directly on the tongue, taste bitter, but when mixed with foods result in an acceptable level of sweetness. However, they do not sweeten the food nearly as much as other artificial sweeteners and for this reason they do not confuse the body's sensory system. Sucralose (Splenda), while not as desirable as stevia or xylitol, is the least disruptive of the other sweeteners.

The health benefits of THE **NO CRAVE** DIET

In addition to weight loss, THE **NO CRAVE** DIET has some tremendously positive effects on your health and risk of disease.

- Lowering cholesterol
- Reducing blood pressure

- Reducing your risk of heart disease
- Preventing and treating Type-2 diabetes

Lowering cholesterol

Hypercholesterolaemia is the term used to define high cholesterol levels in the blood. This is a large contributing factor towards heart disease, as cholesterol is primarily responsible for the blockages that occlude the vessels supplying the heart muscle. Hypercholesterolaemia continues to affect a high percentage of the population, despite the trend towards low-fat products over the past few decades. The reason for this is that the fat you eat only accounts for 18 per cent of your blood fat levels. A low-fat diet will decrease cholesterol levels, but only very slightly. The remaining 82 per cent of fat in your blood is manufactured by your liver from carbohydrates, irrespective of your dietary fat intake. High levels of insulin instruct the liver to increase the production of cholesterol, even from those carbohydrates that are advertised as 'fat and cholesterol free'. They may appear to be the ideal food type for the individual trying to lose weight and lower their cholesterol, but as soon as they are ingested it is a completely different story. THE **NO CRAVE** DIET works on lowering your cholesterol by manipulating 82 per cent of your blood levels rather than 18 per cent.

Hypertension (high blood pressure)

Hypertension is another disease that afflicts a high proportion of the population. Hypertension is defined as an increase in blood pressure above 140 (systolic)/90(diastolic), where normal blood pressure is considered 120/80 or less.

Abnormal hormone levels and altered metabolism that leads to weight gain and food cravings also contribute to high blood pressure. For example, excess insulin directs the kidneys to retain more salt, and when the body retains salt it will always retain extra water. This excess fluid will not only cause bloating and discomfort, but will raise your blood pressure. High cortisol (our stress hormone) tightens blood vessels, which also increases pressure.

THE **NO CRAVE** DIET corrects the hormonal imbalances to bring your blood pressure under control.

Heart disease

High cholesterol is not the only contributing factor towards heart disease. Excess insulin also raises levels of fats called triglycerides, which irritate blood vessels, producing inflammation and damage. This damage leads to 'hardening of the arteries', a major factor in high blood pressure and heart disease. Excess insulin also appears to influence arterial wall thickness.

High levels of the fat messenger hormone leptin promote vessel damage and cardiovascular disease, thickening the arteries, which causes more extensive and complex development of thrombosis-causing plaques. High glucose and insulin levels are known to alter sorbitol metabolism within arterial walls causing further thickening and degeneration. Persistent cortisol production, associated with stress and cravings, adversely affects blood vessels, particularly the coronary arteries of the heart.

THE **NO CRAVE** DIET addresses abnormal levels of insulin, leptin and cortisol, lowering your risk of cardiovascular disease.

Type-2 diabetes

Type-2 diabetes results from insufficient insulin production by the pancreas (the cells become exhausted from overuse) in combination with resistance of tissues to the effects of insulin (the available insulin is no longer effective). Whilst individuals do retain some insulin secretion, they often need oral medication or injected insulin to augment it. Type-2 diabetes results from persistently high blood sugars in susceptible individuals. Chronic hyperglycaemia has an almost toxic effect on the insulin-producing beta cells of the pancreas. This leads to a delayed and decreased insulin secretion in response to high blood glucose. The toxic effect can often be reversed and insulin secretion returned to normal by prolonged stabilisation of blood sugar levels with diet and weight loss.

Type-2 diabetes was almost unheard of in children ten years ago. Related to poor diet and obesity, it was considered a disease of the older age group, hence its original name 'late onset diabetes'. However, its rates have grown exponentially and currently in the UK 9 per cent of boys and 13 per cent of girls between the ages of 5 and 16 have pre-diabetes (the precursor to type-2) or full-blown type-2 diabetes. The UK has the fastest growing rate of childhood type-2 diabetes in the world.

THE **NO CRAVE** DIET not only prevents type-2 diabetes even in the pre-diabetic phase, but it can also often reverse it once established or at the least allow for minimal treatment. Preventing diabetes also greatly reduces the risk of associated health conditions such as cardiovascular disease, kidney failure, loss of eyesight and blocked arteries in the legs.

What has reward got to do with hunger and craving?

We may have just finished a large main course at dinner, but the appearance of the dessert menu almost always warrants a brief perusal. And, despite the fact that we feel pretty full already, the hot chocolate fudge cake still seems very attractive. We know how good it is going to taste, so even though we are clearly not in need of any more nutrition, we order a piece and it does not disappoint!

The decision-making process has little to do with energy balance, satiety peptides or NPY activity in the hypothalamus. It has everything to do with reward. The pleasurable effects of eating that piece of cake have just overridden all the

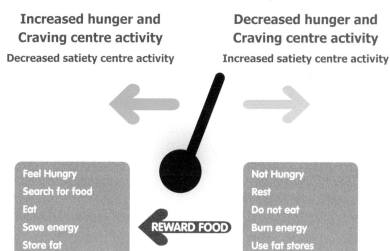

Increased hunger and Craving centre activity
Decreased satiety centre activity

Decreased hunger and Craving centre activity
Increased satiety centre activity

Feel Hungry
Search for food
Eat
Save energy
Store fat

REWARD FOOD

Not Hungry
Rest
Do not eat
Burn energy
Use fat stores

complex interactions that purport to control our food intake. When we eat regular food, the body receives and interprets information about its nutritional content, which is interpreted in terms of our current energy status to determine how much we should ingest. With highly palatable food, the primary message is that received by the reward centre, which encourages us to eat more, regardless of its nutritional value or our energy needs. The brain reward system reinforces behaviour that is of no physiological benefit to the body. It is concerned with feeling good not feeling healthy!

The reward system

The combined effect of a number of neurotransmitters within the brain affects our sense of wellbeing, comfort, satisfaction, calmness and contentment. The most important are serotonin (our natural anti-depressant), the opioid peptides (our natural painkillers), dopamine (our endogenous stimulant) and GABA (gaba-amino-butyric acid – our endogenous sedative). Working together, they act upon our 'reward centre', called the nucleus accumbens (NA), a small area at the base of the forebrain. When acting synergistically they promote production of dopamine within this area, which results in a person feeling satisfied, calm and happy. However, when activity in any of the four systems is impaired and dopamine production in the NA drops, there is a sense of anxiety, incompleteness, agitation and dismay. In an attempt to reverse this, the brain institutes behaviour aimed at restoring 'reward', seeking out food that will increase levels of the appropriate neurotransmitters. This is the basis of 'craving'.

Over the past few years, the role of the reward system in eating behaviour has been studied extensively. Like any other pleasurable activity, eating stimulates certain areas of the brain that make us feel good. It causes release of neurotransmitters known to invoke sensations of happiness, relaxation and comfort. And although the attractiveness of food is somewhat dependent on nutritional status – consider how much better a meal looks or smells when you are hungry – there is certainly evidence that in certain individuals and with prolonged dietary changes, taste becomes the overwhelming influence regardless of the need for more energy.

The four neurotransmitters implicated in the reward process are serotonin, GABA (gaba-amino-butyric acid), the opioid peptides and dopamine.

Serotonin is often called our 'happy hormone' as it induces feelings of calm, personal security, relaxation and confidence. Low levels are associated with depression, and our body feels sluggish, apathetic, sad and weepy. Many anti-depressant drugs work by artificially increasing levels of this chemical in the brain. Serotonin is also involved in the reward system and control of hunger and food intake.

Serotonin is released whenever we consume high-glycaemic carbohydrates (like sugar) and, in particular, chocolate. Serotonin is made from the amino acid tryptophan. Insulin, released in response to a high blood sugar following ingestion of high-glycaemic carbohydrates, removes glucose and some amino acids from the blood. However, it leaves tryptophan, resulting in relatively higher tryptophan levels in the blood and increased production in the brain. This is why, following a high carbohydrate meal, one often feels relaxed and somewhat elated. Similarly, this is why one may crave sweets and starches or other foods that break down quickly into sugar when depressed or in other circumstances when serotonin is low, such as in women before their period. Certain foods are tryptophan-rich, such as turkey – hence the need for that post-Christmas snooze! Unfortunately, a slice of turkey is not nearly as accessible as a chocolate bar when we need that serotonin!

In addition, when people first begin a diet or weight-loss programme, there is an initial drop in serotonin as blood sugar levels drop back to normal. Even though blood sugar levels are only falling to normal and not below normal, the body still senses a change and reacts to this change. During this period, cravings for sweets and starches may exist in an attempt to increase both sugar levels and serotonin. Fortunately, once the body becomes more accustomed to the new blood sugar level, the cravings will dissipate. In chronic stress, not only does the altered carbohydrate metabolism increase the sugar lows and thus the serotonin level, but cortisol also directly reduces serotonin production. Thus, our desire for sweets and starches is even higher.

A diet high in fat also appears to increase serotonin. Medications that increase serotonin levels reduce the desire for fatty foods and studies on stressed animals demonstrate that a high fat content in the diet reduces stress levels by elevating serotonin.

GABA (gaba-amino-butyric acid) is our natural sedative, promoting calm and relaxation. Increased levels of GABA are associated with reduced desire for palatable food, acting to inhibit cravings. Drugs that stimulate GABA receptors in the brain have been investigated and found to reduce appetite and food intake.

The opioid peptides are a group of endogenously produced chemicals in the brain and elsewhere in the body that act in a similar way to the drug morphine. Although initially thought to be only responsible for the control of pain, their role has been expanded to include control of food intake, reward and addiction. High levels are found in the area of the brain called the nucleus accumbens or 'reward centre', which is the principal region implicated in this behaviour. The opioid peptides reinforce the 'coming back for more' behaviour characteristic of overeating.

The opioid peptides selectively promote the ingestion of fatty or sugary foods and, interestingly, do not distinguish between true sugar and artificial sweeteners, indicating that it is the taste rather than the energy content that is driving the behaviour. To compound matters, high fat and sugar diets actually increase the amount of opioid peptides and their receptors, creating a vicious cycle of eating and reward.

Dopamine is the fourth chemical neurotransmitter implicated in the reward system. Eating palatable food increases production of dopamine within the 'reward centre', which leads to a feeling of wellbeing, relaxation and satisfaction. Inadequate dopamine production causes unease or anxiety and results in food-seeking behaviour. However, as with the opioid peptides, when increased production of dopamine is due to ingestion of sweet or palatable food, rather than shutting off the reward centre it encourages it to further increase food intake. After all, if some of this food makes me feel good, more will make me feel even better! This again leads to a vicious cycle of eating and reward.

How reward foods swing the balance

So, with little respect for any of the other control systems, the reward system swings the balance in favour of the 'bad guys'. However well we have our hunger and satiety centres under control, if the reward centre remains active, we will still experience increased appetite, food cravings and have a tendency to put on weight.

Controlling our reward system

Controlling our reward system may prove to be one of the more difficult aspects of any diet. After all, diets are usually a time where you crave a little reward most! However, by careful choice of food, appropriate supplements and techniques to improve mood and reduce stress, our reward system can be made to feel 'good' without the need for chocolate cake! This is yet another reason why **THE NO CRAVE DIET** works.

Questions and answers

Certain times or events seem to produce the most extreme cravings. Using **THE NO CRAVE DIET** will eliminate or considerably ameliorate most of these, but once in a while events out of your control can occur. The following examples explain why the cravings are so intense and what you can do about them.

Question: Why do I always crave a nice greasy bacon sandwich the morning after a night out and a few beers?

Answer:

1. Alcohol causes a low blood sugar, one of the most potent stimulators of food cravings.

2. Alcohol increases levels of our stress hormone, cortisol, which also promotes food cravings.

3. The dehydration caused by alcohol further increases cortisol, as well as making you more hungry.

4. Alcohol lowers levels of dopamine and serotonin, our 'happy hormones', and (as with depression where similar hormonal changes occur) this causes food cravings.

The bacon sarnie provides sugar, calories and the necessary taste stimulus to satisfy the craving – let's face it, no one with a hangover is going to feel like reaching for a soy-protein shake!

No-Crave solution:

During Phase 1 of **THE NO CRAVE DIET**, a night out like this is certainly going to disrupt your metabolic retraining and is not recommended. In Phase 2 it can be tolerated once in a while and the following tips may help reduce its effects on your craving:

1. Have some fibre (celery, carrot, broccoli) and good fat (flax oil, unsalted walnuts, omega-enriched dip) before you head out.

2. Have some food with your drinks that is high in protein.

3. Drink one glass of water for each alcoholic drink and one pint before bed.

4. Have a protein breakfast such as a smoothie or an egg-white omelette ready for when you get up.

Question: Relationship problems always increase my cravings, what can I do?

Answer:

Food cravings almost always rear their ugly heads during times of stress, but there are a few stressors that seem particularly effective at stimulating them. A relationship problem such as a break-up with a boyfriend or girlfriend is certainly one of those times. It has been shown that love, or simply being in the presence of a person we are attracted to, increases dopamine, our reward chemical messenger in the brain. During and after a break-up dopamine levels fall and the reward centre goes into withdrawal, encouraging you to seek dopamine-inducing comfort foods such as sweets and fats. Our cortisol rises and levels of serotonin, the happy hormone that balances our cravings for chocolates and sweets, falls. The combination of changes in these three chemical messengers spells disaster for our hunger and craving centre.

No-Crave solution:

You may have already eaten the double fudge, macadamia nut, caramel swirl ice cream and washed it down with a few drinks with your girlfriends whilst running over all the benefits of being single. Just put that one very large cheat behind you and move on with your diet and your life.

You know there is a temporary stressor in your life that will be present in your daily thoughts for the next few weeks or so, so you need to arm yourself for when those cravings hit:

1. The good news is that we know the two main chemical messengers involved and we know how to boost them back up without your boyfriend or the ice cream. L-tyrosine and 5-HTP can be taken in capsule form two to three times a day to help support and rebalance the production and use of these messengers. It is almost like a 'boyfriend in a bottle' – if only it were that easy!

2. Next we need to keep protein treats in chocolate flavour around everywhere, a bar in your purse, protein powder in your desk at work, some of the home-made protein cookie dough in the freezer at home. Arm yourself with treats. It is just as important to keep ready-washed and chopped veggies and protein sources such as cooked chicken or beef in the fridge.

3. Booking yourself a massage or facial and generally pampering yourself will also stimulate those feel-good messengers and prevent cravings for food from sabotaging your diet.

4. Starting a new exercise programme will reduce cravings, stimulate your happy hormones and, along with your diet, get you in great shape.

5. Write some new diet commandments to include why you want to look good for yourself and to show your ex what they're missing!

Question: Why do my cravings always increase before my period?

Answer:

During the week before our menstrual cycle many of us can be a little more demanding or slightly less rational. Well, the same hormones responsible for those behaviours (oestrogen and progesterone) block the use of serotonin (our happy hormone) and increase cortisol (our stress hormone). Of course, we all know it's coming every single month, so there really shouldn't be any surprise when we have a sudden desire to reach for the box of chocolate brownies on the way to the supermarket checkout. But for some reason, on the 24th or 25th day of each cycle we are confounded by the overpowering pull towards the chocolate aisle and our seeming lack of control over it.

Apart from visiting your doctor, testing and rebalancing your ratio of oestrogen to progesterone, detoxifying your liver and barricading yourself in your room for one week each month, there are a few simple tricks you can use to fool your body into thinking it has already had the chocolate, and begin to slowly balance the hormones responsible for this annoying monthly ritual in the first place.

No-Crave solution:

1. The number-one priority here is chocolate – so get some, just make it protein chocolate. Go back to your double-chocolate-crunch protein bars, satisfy the serotonin fix with chocolate, yet stabilise your blood sugars at the same time to prevent a hypoglycaemic crash that would stimulate another chocolate craving half an hour later. If the cravings are extremely intense, supplementing with 5-HTP and 100mg of vitamin B6 daily will support increased serotonin production.

2. Omega-3 fatty acids, such as flax oil or fish oils, are also very useful. Taking these daily will balance the ratio of serotonin to cortisol as well as increase dopamine, the relaxing and reward messenger of the brain.

3. Magnolia flower is another useful weapon here. Not only will magnolia greatly reduce the production of cortisol, but it will also begin to rebalance the levels of oestrogen and progesterone in the body, back to a more even ratio with fewer pre-menstrual symptoms.

4. Chart your cycle and, more importantly, chart the week before so you can stock up on your PMS armoury and win the battle against your hormones.

Question: Why do I always crave more when I am out enjoying myself?

Answer:

It is Saturday afternoon and your football team has made it through to the FA Cup final. You are meeting your mates at the pub to watch the game. You know the pints will be flowing. You are not depressed; serotonin and dopamine are high, in fact higher than normal. You do not feel overwhelmed or stressed so your cortisol should be stable. So there should be no reason for your cravings to appear.

Unfortunately your stress system does not know the difference between a positive and a negative stress. The excitement of the game, win or lose, is interpreted in just the same way as a final exam or a job interview. And once the stress hormones start, the effect on your hunger and cravings is just the same. Your brain will react by searching out something to calm it down and alcohol, believe it or not, has a depressing action within the nervous system. In addition to increasing your craving for beer, the stress hormones will encourage you to order the bar snack with the highest carbohydrate and fat content.

No-Crave solution:

1. Knowing the afternoon's entertainment will increase your stress hormones, take a capsule or two of milk peptides or green tea extract before you go.

2. Have some fibre (celery, carrot, broccoli) and good fat (flax oil, unsalted walnuts, omega-enriched dip) before you head out. It's even better if you can eat a No-Crave meal before you go.

3. Order some chicken with veggies and dip at the beginning of the game so you have them right there and ready to gnaw on when the craving hits.

4. Drink a glass of water for every alcoholic drink you have. This will make you feel more full, will enable you to drink less, will reduce the dehydrating effects of the alcohol and you'll still be able to celebrate.

Planning for a crave-inducing event

Unexpected or planned events can put extra stress on your hunger and craving centre. While THE **NO CRAVE** DIET will help you deal with most of these, having a few extra tricks up your sleeve is always useful.

Friends ask you for drinks after work unexpectedly

It is Thursday at 4:30 p.m., you have had a long day at work, your energy reserves are low and you have had nothing to eat since lunch. You have your carefully planned No-Crave dinner at home, curried chicken and vegetables with salad, waiting for you in the fridge. A friend pops into your office and tells you that a group of colleagues are going around the corner in half an hour to grab a quick drink and review tomorrow's meeting agenda. You know your food options will be limited, and that once that first sip of beer or wine passes your lips your desire to keep drinking and munch on crisps will rise. The good news is that you have time to prepare.

1. Tell your 'buddy' about the event and see if they can go with you.

2. Drink three large glasses of water to fill your stomach. Then take one capsule of l-tyrosine, letting it dissolve slowly in your mouth to help suppress those craving centres and balance the reward centres.

3. Let everyone know beforehand that you will not be having any alcohol. Take a protein bar in case the meeting runs late so you at least have some version of protein to nibble on until you get home.

4. Read your diet commandments before you leave.

5. Take a pen and paper to write some notes as a distraction.

6. Put a reminder of your end-of-week reward in your pocket and remember that a cheat puts it out of reach.

The business lunch meeting

Your weekly Wednesday lunch meeting is normally catered with a variety of No-Crave-friendly choices such as quiche, tuna and veggies or chicken Caesar salad. Today, however, someone else ordered and the choice includes pizza, sandwiches and muffins.

Before giving in and convincing yourself that you really have no choice, remember that in the early days in your No-Crave programme just one bite of that greasy, carbohydrate-heavy pizza can stimulate days of further craving. A few days into **THE NO CRAVE DIET** you wouldn't even think about these foods when they are not in front of you. Just because they are, don't give in.

1. Think about what 'emergency' No-Crave foods you have in the office such as a protein bar or protein powder (such as vanilla protein powder) in your desk, or some cottage or ricotta cheese in the fridge. Have these instead of the pizza, adding as much salad as you like from the lunch table.

2. Drink some water.

3. Take an l-glutamine.

4. Do one of your deep-breathing exercises and try to arrive late at the lunch so most of the food is gone – you know there'll be plenty of salad left over!

5. Scan your food choices for the best possible option. Look for chicken, egg or tuna sandwiches and leave the surrounding bread. Fill your plate with veggies and salad if available.

Your co-workers bring you a cake for your birthday

It is your birthday and you have already told your family you don't want a birthday cake. If they insist on something, suggest as a treat some 70 per cent dark chocolate to have one square at a time when you wish, or perhaps a special bottle of wine. You know these foods are not allowed during Phase 1 of **THE NO CRAVE DIET**, but it is your birthday after all and you are allowing yourself a cheat knowing that at home you can at least balance things out by combining them with a large portion of protein.

Unfortunately at lunchtime, despite protests from your 'buddy', your friends surprise you with a special birthday cake.

1. It is unlikely to work but you could try thanking them, say you are not feeling great but will take it home to share with your family.

2. Grab the knife first and cut off a large piece for everyone in the office, even those you are not particularly friendly with. This will remove your temptation and make you highly popular!

3. Take a very small portion for yourself while you chat.

4. Make sure that if you do have some cake you have some protein (part of a protein bar, a protein shake, chicken or cottage cheese from the fridge) at the same time, or as soon as the get-together is over. Remember, by combining the protein with your cheat food, you will slow down the delivery of the cheat food into the blood and therefore store less of the food as fat, and decrease the chances of this food causing further food cravings later on in the day.

Case studies
KT is a fifteen-year-old female

At the age of twelve she started putting on a significant amount of weight. She spent several nights each week eating pizza, drinking fizzy drinks with her friends, playing video games and eating biscuits between meals. She found she could not control her eating, and would often head down to the kitchen in the middle of night when her parents were sleeping to get a snack. KT became very unhappy with her weight, and her parents became concerned when her doctor mentioned that her blood sugar levels were rising and she may end up with diabetes. After trying to cut out the snacks and treats, KT found her cravings intensified, leading to even more food between meals and at night.

KT's mother brought her into my office and, after examining her and going through her diet, it was evident that KT's brain chemistry was completely controlling her food behaviour. Once I had explained the problem and why she needed to lose weight for her health, KT started **THE NO CRAVE DIET**. She learned temptation therapies that would support her diet and began an exercise programme. I also suggested temporary supplementation with magnolia flower, 5-HTP, a multi-B-vitamin complex and l-carnosine.

KT began to lose weight quite rapidly, dropping on average about three pounds per week in the first month, followed with two pounds a week for the next two months. Six months later, KT has kept the weight off, her blood sugars are normal, and she has joined the football team at school. She no longer craves food between meals and has dessert or treats only on special occasions or with friends – this by her choice, for she reports 'not needing them any more'. When she does have them, she is quickly satisfied after small amounts and never asks for a second helping.

LG is a 31-year-old female

LG gave birth to her first child eight months ago. She found that while pregnant she consumed more carbohydrates than ever before in order to control her nausea in the first trimester. The nausea greatly subsided in the second trimester, but she then found she was addicted to carbohydrates, mostly in the form of muffins, pasta and bread. She became irritable and cranky if she did not have them at every meal, but more importantly she could not stop obsessively thinking about them until she satisfied her craving. After the birth of her son, the cravings continued. She desperately tried to ignore them, but they kept taking her back to the cupboard or fridge after each meal.

When LG came to see me she was still breast-feeding so I modified Phase 1 of the diet. We did not completely take away all grains and starches from her diet. Rather, we kept them in at breakfast, but ensured that she consumed a larger amount of protein at that meal to balance the grains (in the form of whole-grain toast or oatmeal), along with her 'good carbs' of fruit or vegetables. Lunch and dinner included appropriate amounts of protein combined only with fruit and vegetables. We also added milk peptides, malic acid, essential fatty acids and calcium–magnesium to her daily regime, as they were safe during breast-feeding.

LG reported a significant reduction in cravings within 24 hours, and by the third day, she did not even need her toast, and often added more vegetables or fruit to her breakfast to maintain the extra carbohydrate needed for breast-feeding. She dropped just over two pounds per week while breast-feeding. We kept a close watch on blood sugars and ketones in her urine to make sure that all her levels were normal, and that she wasn't starving herself or her baby. Four months later, LG has lost all the weight gained during her pregnancy and has dropped down to a clothing size that she has not been in for years.

Susan is a 45-year-old mother of three

She has struggled for years trying to lose what she thought was extra baby weight that lingered predominantly around her waist. Every time Susan started a diet she was very diligent for one week to ten days. She followed all instructions to the letter, and felt great. She started to see results, was less bloated and had much better energy. However, there were always treats in her house for her children. During what she called 'moments of weakness' she would have a bite or small amount of a biscuit, a mouthful of ice cream or simply finish what was left on one of children's dessert plates. This little bit of 'cheat' stimulated further desire to fill up on more sweets. For some reason she could not stop eating the treats and sweets after tasting them, and this would completely sabotage her weight-loss programme.

Following my evaluation I found that both her dopamine and serotonin levels were low. This led to feelings of deprivation and dissatisfaction, so that once given a small taste of 'satisfaction' from treat food, the feelings could not be ignored. Her body chemically desired more and more. Her previous weight-loss diets were far too low in protein, which meant that her blood-sugar levels were fairly unstable despite her so-called healthy choices of bran and brown rice to accompany her vegetables and fruit.

Once I started Susan on THE **NO CRAVE** DIET and began natural supplementation with l-tyrosine, 5-HTP and l-glutamine, her food cravings and desire to snack were absent even when she did decide to taste some of her children's cake. She was able to retrain the communication centres in her brain and teach them not to have 'out of control' reactions to food. She has put more balance back into her life, is not controlled by hunger and cravings and, one and a half years since we met, her weight loss and cravings are both stable.

Mark is a 38-year-old financial planner

He works for a rather demanding and abrupt boss who continually places demands upon him. There are many nights Mark lies awake worrying about his career, his workload and whether or not he will live up to his boss's expectations. Before starting this job Mark never had a weight problem. He came to see me complaining of uncontrollable food cravings, having gained ten pounds over the past four months, due to food binges following stress.

Mark maintained a very balanced diet and healthy exercise regime. However, every time his boss became angry with him, or made unrealistic demands upon him, Mark would invariably turn to chocolate bars or crisps to 'soothe' or calm his emotions. Before he knew it, he was eating these foods frequently, which only made his body more tired, more stressed, and spurred on more food cravings.

I quickly discovered that Mark's stress (adrenal) glands were extremely taxed and had an exaggerated response to even the smallest stressors. This in turn led him to seek out treats to block or mask the side effects of the elevated stress hormones. Mark started THE NO CRAVE DIET as well as No-Crave anti-stress therapies including natural supplementation with milk peptides, GABA and a multi-B-vitamin complex, and lifestyle techniques such as regular massage, deep breathing and yoga.

After only two weeks on the programme, Mark reported a complete absence of food cravings. He was eating healthily, felt calmer, had more energy and was more productive at work. His weight was returning to normal, allowing him to progress rapidly into Phase 2 of the diet.

Mary is a 37-year-old female

Mary came to my office wishing to lose weight. She explained that despite eating well and exercising regularly, she had continued to gain, particularly around the mid-section. I went over her diet and exercise regime, tested her for thyroid and growth-hormone insufficiencies, and found no particular problems. Her diet was balanced, with protein at each meal, good quantities of vegetables and salads, a small amount of fruit and little to no high-glycaemic foods. She maintained an exercise regime of forty-five minutes to an hour of cardio five times a week, with two to three days of weight training. Despite her admirable attempts at positive lifestyle choices, she had continued to gain weight. Frustrated, she tried several over-the-counter diet supplements, with little to no success.

During the interview we discovered that she never gave herself any relaxation time, except when on holiday. And, whenever she was on holiday, she reported losing significant weight quickly and a substantial decrease in bloating. This was despite a poorer diet, decreased exercise and increased alcohol intake. On her return home the weight was rapidly regained.

The fact that she consistently lost weight on holiday and gained weight at home, independent of diet and exercise, led me to think that stress was the main factor responsible for her unstable body weight. Mary is a lawyer working long hours, has two young children and little time for herself. She used exercise as her only stress-management technique, but this was often performed in a rush and with her mind preoccupied with closing statements for an upcoming case.

Mary started **THE NO CRAVE DIET**, some massage therapy, some yoga and deep breathing, a course of magnolia extract, and vitamin B complex. Two weeks later she had lost four pounds and overall felt much more relaxed. After one month she had lost the seven pounds she had wanted to lose and has subsequently maintained this weight.

Mary now realises the importance of keeping her stress levels down, and although her career does not always allow her as much free time as she would like, she makes a point of increasing her deep breathing, yoga and cortisol-reducing supplements when life starts to get more hectic. She has now learned the balance of lifestyle factors that work well for her, allowing her body to function at the capacity she needs without causing damage.

Supplement information
Basic Terms

The term 'nutritional supplement' includes vitamins, minerals, enzymes and coenzymes, essential fatty acids, amino acids and herbs.

Vitamins

Any constituents in the diet other than protein, fat, carbohydrate and inorganic salts that are necessary for normal growth and physical activity. They must be obtained from external sources, and a deficiency may cause diseases, depending on the vitamin.

Minerals

Essentially any inorganic substance found in the earth. Like vitamins, minerals must be taken in from an outside source and are necessary for proper bodily maintenance and growth. Minerals can be divided into two categories. 'Macrominerals' are those the body needs in larger doses of milligrams or even grams. This includes such minerals as calcium, magnesium, phosphorus and potassium. 'Trace' minerals are those required in much smaller amounts, in micrograms. This category includes iodine, selenium and chromium, for example.

Enzymes and coenzymes

Vitamins and minerals are essential components of enzymes and coenzymes. Enzymes are substances that stimulate different biochemical reactions in the body. Coenzymes aid the enzymes in this function. With proper nutritional supplementation, we can support certain enzymatic pathways to perform optimally, thereby speeding up certain reactions. If an enzyme is lacking a vitamin or mineral, it cannot function optimally and the process is slowed or halted. We must therefore ensure adequate nutrient supplementation to accentuate certain bodily functions.

Essential fatty acids

Most people try to stay away from fatty foods, and for the most part this is a wise decision. However, there are some fats that are actually beneficial – indeed, essential to the body. Most people are approximately 70 to 80 per cent deficient in essential fatty acids. The symptoms of a low dietary intake of essential fats are fatigue, dry skin and hair, constipation, depression, bloating and arthritis.

Amino acids

These are the component parts of protein molecules and are therefore needed for tissue repair, enzyme reactions, nerve and muscle function, and recovery. Nonessential amino acids can be manufactured by the body, while essential ones need to be part of our diet.

Herbs

Herbal supplementation is the use of botanicals or natural plants as therapeutic agents. Over 70 per cent of prescription drugs are based on plant formulas, so by using the original plant we can often achieve a similar result. Botanicals or herbs will often have the same physiological effect as a drug. They will bind into the same receptors and produce a similar outcome. The difference lies in the strength. Generally, herbal medicine is much weaker, ranging from one hundredth to one thousandth the strength of its pharmaceutical equivalent. Thus the natural medications require more time to have an effect. However, the benefit is that their side effects are generally minimal. Once again, by combining both forms of therapy, we can achieve a maximal effect with minimal side effects. This is done by decreasing the dose of pharmaceuticals and enhancing the therapeutic effect with natural supplementation.

Supplement Safety

Supplements, although natural, can have side effects and interactions with other medications (both natural and pharmaceutical). So check the label and, if you are concerned, discuss with your doctor, particularly if you are already on medication. Always inform any doctor or surgeon who treats you about every medication you are taking, natural or otherwise.

	L-Glutamine	Hoodia	Carnosine	Green Tea	5-HTP	GABA	CLA	L-Tyrosine	Inulin
Reduces Cravings									
Short term	X	X							
Long term			X	X	X	X	X	X	
Reduces Appetite		X	X						X
Reduces Stress				X	X	X			
Stabilises Blood Sugar									X
Increases Fat Burning		X		X			X		

	Melatonin	Calcium	Magnesium	Malic Acid	Garcinia cambogia	Citrus aurantium	Milk Peptide	Magnolia	Chromium
Reduces Cravings									
Short term									
Long term		X	X						
Reduces Appetite									
Reduces Stress	X						X	X	
Stabilises Blood Sugar	X								X
Increases Fat Burning				X	X	X			

L-glutamine

When you are hit with a food craving, particularly a sweet one, this simple amino acid can help eradicate it within thirty seconds. When we see a food we desire, or think about a food we may wish to eat, our salivary glands begin to release digestive juices that interact with our taste buds, and send a message to our brain to further stimulate the urge to eat this food. L-glutamine interacts with the same taste receptors on the tongue to extinguish that message to the brain within seconds. If you feel unable to resist the biscuit or brownie you desire, open up a 500mg capsule of l-glutamine and put it directly on the tongue with a sip of water. Hold it in the mouth for about thirty seconds, and then swallow. You will be surprised how quickly the craving subsides. L-glutamine is also great for muscle and bowel repair, so you will also be doing your body a favour! You can easily intake up to 5000mg a day if you need to, but remember, the longer you go without a specific type of food treat, the less you will desire it.

Dose

One 500mg capsule twice a day. To stop a craving open a 500mg capsule on your tongue and hold it in your mouth for thirty seconds.

Any side effects?

None reported.

Green tea

Buddhist monks originally brought green tea to Japan from China, where it was quickly embraced by the Japanese as a soothing, calming drink and was found to have numerous health benefits. It comes from the same plant as traditional black tea, *Camellia sinesis*, and is produced by steaming and drying fresh tea leaves at elevated temperatures in order to keep the active ingredients intact. Green tea has six times more antioxidant activity than black tea.

Green tea boosts metabolism, increases calorie burning and promotes fat utilisation. Unlike other dietary stimulants such as caffeine, green tea increases metabolism without any increase in heart rate or blood pressure.

Green tea extract also acts on certain receptors in the gut to help reduce feelings of hunger and food cravings. From a health viewpoint, green tea contains powerful antioxidants and has six times more antioxidant activity than regular black tea.

Dose

300mg of green tea extract twice a day on an empty stomach. (Alternatively, you could drink green tea as an infusion, but this is much weaker than the supplement form, the dose is hard to control and the added caffeine may cause side effects.)

Any side effects?

Very few side effects have been seen with green tea extracts or the tea itself. However, as they both contain caffeine, if you are highly sensitive to this ingredient, you may experience palpitations, increased sweating or anxiety similar to drinking a cup of coffee. The tea leaves themselves contain far more caffeine than the supplement pills, so if you are concerned try the supplement before the tea itself.

5-HTP

5-HTP, or 5-hydroxytryptophan is a close relative of serotonin, our happy hormone, and therefore aids in wellbeing, relaxation and stress relief. Chocolate and sweets make you feel good as they promote release of serotonin and 5-HTP in the brain. This feel-good effect is what you crave. So by taking a natural supplement you cut out the cake-eating step and still get to feel good! Taken during times of stress 5-HTP exerts a calming effect, improving relaxation and sleep.

Dose

For general relief of anxiety, 50 to 100mg twice a day is sufficient.

Any side effects?

Although 5-HTP already exists in the body naturally, occasional upset stomach or increased abnormal euphoria can be seen at high doses (200mg twice a day). If you are already taking medication, particularly antidepressants, then 5-HTP should be avoided.

L-tyrosine

Tyrosine, also called l-tyrosine, is an amino acid vital to the production of many hormones and neurotransmitters in the body that deal with weight, food cravings and energy levels.

When taken as a supplement tyrosine triggers the release of cholecystokinin in the gut. This appetite-suppressing hormone is also released when we eat fatty or savoury foods. It stimulates the satiety centre in the brain, leading to feelings of satisfaction, fullness and decreasing the desire to consume more food. Taking the tyrosine supplement produces the same effect without the fat intake.

Tyrosine also is crucial for the production of thyroid hormones, which are essential for maintaining a healthy metabolism and burning off excess calories. Stress can reduce the amount of active thyroid hormone in the body, an effect counteracted by tyrosine.

Dose
500mg to 1000mg twice a day without food.
Any side effects?
None reported.

Milk peptides

These natural casein extracts from milk help to decrease the excess release of stress hormones, calming your overactive HPA axis – the stress-response pathway. By adding this supplement to your regimen, you will be less likely to get overwhelmed by the day-to-day stressors leading to an inadvertent trip to the fridge. Mother knew best when she said a hot milk before bed will help you relax and sleep!

Milk contains a high concentration of peptides or chains of amino acids. The tryptic hydrolysate decapeptide is one particular sequence of amino acids that is ten units or amino acids long. It is found in milk and has been shown to possess strong anxiolytic properties. This may account for the soothing effect mother's milk has on the child, beyond satisfying the stressful situation of being hungry.

In adults with high levels of pepsin, the small amount of this peptide found in normal milk is rapidly broken down. However, by increasing the ingested concentration above pepsin capacity, adults will also absorb some of the anxiolytic decapeptide.

Like many anti-anxiety drugs, tryptic hydrolysate decapeptide specifically binds into the GABA receptor. The GABA receptors are responsible for negative feedback or inhibition in the nervous system and reduce stimulation of the HPA axis, decreasing the stress response and increasing relaxation and calmness. Unlike the pharmaceutical drugs used to produce this effect, use of tryptic hydrolysate decapeptide is not accompanied by sedation.

Dose

100 to 200mg twice a day, but you can take an extra 50mg when feeling sad or anxious.

Any side effects?

Those with a casein allergy should avoid it, but it is fine for those allergic to lactose or whey.

CLA

CLA, or conjugated linoleic acid, is an omega-6 fatty acid, one of the three essential fatty acids (the others are omega-3 and omega-9). CLA is best known for its role in weight loss, whereby it prevents the breakdown of muscle during dieting or strenuous exercise programmes, and forces the body to only use fat stores.

CLA also helps to prevent leptin resistance, allowing this important fat-signalling hormone to get its message through to the brain. Leptin tells the brain we have had enough to eat and have sufficient fat stores, and resistance to its effects promotes hunger and food craving. Finally, CLA displaces saturated fats from the liver for better insulin regulation, cholesterol control and liver health.

Dose

500 to 1000mg twice a day.

Any side effects?

You can get looser stools if you take too much, but this is generally just a softer stool not crampy diarrhoea.

Hoodia

Hoodia gordonii is a cactus plant native to certain semi-desert regions in Africa. It has gained great notoriety of late and is touted as the new natural-wonder weight-loss pill. Native Africans have been using this plant for centuries to help them through their long treks across arid land with little to no food. Not only does this simple cactus decrease their appetite, it also reduces their desire for and thoughts about food. In addition it produces a general sense of wellbeing and alertness without stimulation. Scientists feel that hoodia may mimic the effect glucose has on the brain, thus promoting satiety without the actual intake of calories. Research on animals and humans has shown that hoodia has the ability to reduce appetite and food intake by up to 50 per cent.

Dose

400 to 800mg twice a day, between meals.

Any side effects?

None reported.

Inulin fibre

Inulin fibre is a 100 per cent natural fibre product derived from chicory root. Although technically a carbohydrate, tough bonds linking the molecules render it indigestible by the human gut. It attracts water within the stomach making you feel full and reducing appetite.

An additional benefit is that this complex non-digestible carbohydrate is slowly metabolised in the colon, being fermented by colonic bacteria to produce fatty acids and lactate that the body can use for long-term energy. This slow method of metabolism has the advantage of providing essentially no sugar load (the glycaemic index is zero) while preventing hunger due to lack of fuel. Inulin also appears to stabilise blood sugar and reduce production of bad low-density fats.

Dose

1 teaspoon to 1 tablespoon twice a day.

Any side effects?

May cause flatulence.

Garcinia cambogia

Garcinia cambogia is a fruit grown in southern India that contains a compound known as HCA or hydroxycitric acid. This acid has been clinically proven to reduce weight through two different mechanisms. First, it inhibits lipogenesis, the formation of fat from the food we eat. This process occurs without altering protein metabolism, thereby preserving lean body tissue or muscle for maximal fat-burning potential.

Secondly, *garcinia cambogia* is an appetite suppressant. HCA stimulates a feeling of satiety and satisfaction earlier in a meal, thereby decreasing the amount of food consumed as well as cravings for further food intake.

Dose

350 to 500mg twice a day between meals.

Any side effects?

You may notice an increase in body heat or warmth due to faster fat burning.

Citrus aurantium

Citrus aurantium, otherwise known as bitter orange, has a thermogenic effect that enables the body to mobilise fat more effectively. It helps to carry fat from where it is stored in the body to the mitochondria or fat-burning power units within cells. *Citrus aurantium* also helps to improve the overall metabolic rate, thereby increasing the actual rate at which fat is used. However, this increase is safe as it will only support or stimulate the metabolic rate up to its optimal level. It will not increase the metabolism above normal levels, a dangerous effect of supplements like ephedra.

Dose

150mg twice a day between meals.

Any side effects?

Increased bodily heat or warmth due to faster fat burning.

Malic acid

Malic acid is a natural fruit acid that also exists in every cell in the body. It is crucial for many bodily functions. This simple natural supplement just may be a magic bullet when it comes to weight loss. Malic acid is a powerful antioxidant that decreases oxidation and inflammation. It stimulates a chemical system in the cells of the body, which increases the rate of your metabolism and fat burning. This means you burn more calories and fat even at rest!

Low levels of ATP are seen in overweight individuals and those with low energy levels. Increasing the activity of our cell's powerhouse mitochondria not only uses more fat but also improves energy and performance. Malic acid improves the efficiency of the pathways that burn fat and produce ATP (the uncoupled protein (UCP) pathway), thereby promoting weight loss.

Dose

500mg twice a day.

Any side effects?

As malate is always combined with magnesium, and magnesium is a natural laxative, a few people may experience a softening of the stools. Otherwise no known side effects.

L-carnosine

L-carnosine is a naturally occurring short protein found in the brain, muscle and heart cells where it acts as an antioxidant. Adequate levels are also necessary to minimise the impact of stress on brain cells.

This amino acid is one of the newer anti-ageing supplements to help decrease free radicals, wrinkles and collagen breakdown. However, it also reduces levels of the hunger messenger responsible for you feeling hungry between meals. Good for the initial stages of any diet when levels of the hunger messenger are particularly high.

Dose

500mg twice a day on an empty stomach.

Any side effects?

None known.

Chromium

Chromium is a mineral that was first nicknamed the 'glucose tolerance factor'. It is now known that chromium is not a glucose factor itself, but rather an active factor in blood-sugar control mechanisms. Chromium functions quite intimately with insulin in the uptake of glucose from the blood. Its main role is to help insulin function properly so that it only takes the appropriate amount of glucose from the blood at any given time.

There are several forms of chromium including polynicotinate, chloride, picolinate and chromium-enriched yeasts. Most studies have been performed on chromium picolinate and therefore this is most commonly used form.

Dose

200 micrograms (mcg) a day.

Any side effects?

Kidney irritation at doses above 600mcg a day when taken for prolonged periods of time, such as four weeks.

Melatonin

Melatonin, produced by the tiny pineal gland in the brain, is our body's sleeping hormone. It regulates the daily rhythms of our body, not just our sleep–wake cycle. In addition, melatonin has now been shown to play a role in metabolism, body weight, diabetes and insulin resistance. Melatonin production significantly declines as we age, and this decline is associated with increased deposition of fat, particularly around our abdominal organs, a location associated with significant health risks.

Supplementation with melatonin not only reduces stress and improves our sleep, it helps regulate insulin and leptin, stabilising our blood sugar and increasing our metabolism. It may also help regulate our body's 'set-point' for weight, reducing fat deposition in our mid-section.

Dose

3mg at night.

Any side effects?

May cause a little drowsiness for two to three hours after ingestion.

GABA

Our emotions are controlled by the activity of certain chemical messengers in the brain. These messengers are called neurotransmitters and they mediate signals between nerve cells, allowing communication not only between different areas of the brain but also with the spinal cord and organs throughout the body. Effective functioning requires an adequate supply of neurotransmitters, and disruption in their delicate balance leads to moodiness and overemotional behaviour.

GABA (gamma-amino-butyric acid) is the second most common neurotransmitter in the brain, active at 40 per cent of all synapses. It is also the primary inhibitory neurotransmitter. GABA's primary role is to dampen excessive excitatory neuronal messages, with the vast majority of neurons continually receiving low-level GABA stimulation, a phenomenon known as tonic inhibition. The calming and anxiolytic properties of the benzodiazepine drugs such as diazepam (Valium) are produced by their ability to potentiate GABA activity.

Supplementation with GABA is beneficial in the regulation and restoration of balance in the central nervous system. This is a safe and effective way of promoting relaxation and reducing symptoms associated with stress, allowing the body to relax, calm down and feel balanced.

Dose

500mg twice a day.

Any side effects?

No known side effects but I have found about 1 per cent of people may feel as if they had had a glass of wine.

Magnolia bark extract

Magnolia bark or *Magnolia officinalis* is a traditional Chinese herb. In Chinese medicine it has been used since 100AD for treating what the Chinese refer to as blocked or stagnated qi (pronounced 'chee'). Qi in Chinese medicine is the energy and life force of the body. When qi is blocked it causes symptoms such as low energy, emotional distress or anxiety, digestive complaints, dizziness and alterations in the sleep cycle. In Western medicine this would equal stress and fatigue.

In both forms of medicine magnolia bark is used as a general anti-stress and anti-anxiety herb. Magnolia bark contains many different therapeutic compounds. The two most often used and studied are the biphenols called magnolol and honokiol. However, other ingredients such as beta-eudesmol, and bornyl acetate have also proven to have great therapeutic potential. All of these are the ingredients that possess anxiolytic or anxiety-reducing properties.

The stress-relieving effects of magnolia are quite clear. They have often been equated to that of a benzodiazepine such as Valium, a pharmaceutical anti-anxiety drug. However, benzodiazepines cause sedation, which makes daytime activities quite difficult. The magnolia bark extracts do not have any of the sedating or sleepy qualities. Although most people do sleep more soundly when taking them, it is an indirect effect through cortisol reduction rather than direct sedation. In this way, magnolia becomes a very important agent in the treatment of panic disorders, anxiety and stress.

Dose

For the average 140 to 150-pound adult, 500mg of extract twice a day on an empty stomach.

Any side effects?

No side effects have been seen with magnolia bark extract. In some people who are used to high stress, fatigue may ensue for the first couple of days. It is important to note that this is not sedation, but rather a return to normal energy levels, not the falsely elevated energy levels we often refer to as an adrenaline high.

Passionflower

Passionflower (*Passiflora incarnata*) has been used medicinally for centuries, as a sedative by the Aztecs and as an antispasmodic and anxiolytic stress reliever by Europeans. Some of the first clinical studies were performed in Italy, where passionflower was observed to decrease in brain excitation and prolonged sleeping hours with no adverse side effects. In France, a multi-centre study of anxious patients was carried out to evaluate a plant extract containing botanicals including passionflower. The plant extract produced significantly greater improvement in symptoms than the placebo.

A further double-blind, randomised, controlled study in 2001 compared passionflower directly to a pharmaceutical anti-anxiety drug, Oxazepam, in 36 patients with anxiety disorder. There was no significant difference between the groups with respect to anxiety reduction, but the passionflower group demonstrated far less sedation and impairment of daily function.

Dose

500mg of dried herb twice a day. Passionflower is most frequently prescribed in combination with other herbs.

Any side effects?

While drowsiness or sedation is rare, it can occur in some individuals in higher doses (over 750mg per day). If you are affected, caution is recommended when driving or operating machinery.

Calcium–magnesium at a 1:1 ratio

These simple minerals help maximise the fat-burning process in the body.

Dose

500mg of each twice a day, with or without food.

Any side effects?

Calcium is a natural constipator, and magnesium is a natural laxative. For those with very loose bowel movements, magnesium at this dose can further soften the stools. If that is the case, then halve the magnesium dose, but do not take the calcium on its own.

Multi-B vitamin

B vitamins have been coined the anti-stress vitamins, and with good reason. B6 and B12 help to increase the production of serotonin, our happy hormone. They also lower cortisol, our stress hormone. B5 is used in the fat-burning process and B1 and B3 are used to decrease cholesterol and fat build-up. They are recommended for PMS, headaches and mood swings, all of which can weaken one's willpower and lead to food cravings.

Dose

100mg of a multi-B vitamin containing Bs 1, 3, 5, 6 and 12, to be taken with food.

Any side effects?

Safe, but will turn urine bright yellow. Vitamin B3 can cause a harmless flushing of the skin with a feeling of heat and itchiness. This can be avoided by taking a combination version called niacinamide, rather than pure B3 which is called niacin – just check the label or ask.

Useful contacts and suppliers

Where to buy supplements

- Holland and Barrett
- Sainsburys
- Boots

Your local health food store and pharmacy can also order in natural supplements on request from natural supplement companies such as:

Some reputable brands

- Holland and Barrett
- Solaray
- AOR
- TwinLab
- Quest
- Pharmanex

Online websites that will deliver to the UK, or have present distribution in the UK

- www.pkrhealth.ca – Dr Kendall-Reed's clinic can ship out any of the required supplements anywhere in the world
- www.hollandandbarrett.com
- www.aor.ca
- www.twinlab.com
- www.questvitamins.com
- www.pharmanex.com
- www.obcusa.co.uk/home.php (stocks Go-Lean protein cereal)

Penny rates egg white as the best source of protein for no-cravers, and free range liquid egg white in cartons was recently being promoted as the new superfood to try. This is the supplier: www.twochicks.co.uk. They have lots of info and recipe suggestions on their site.

Glossary

α-MSH: The major satiety or anti-hunger messenger in the brain.

Adipokine: A messenger or hormone produced by fat cells e.g. leptin.

Adipose tissue: Your fat deposits.

Adrenal glands: Glands that sit above each kidney and produce hormone messengers including cortisol.

AGRP: (Agouti-related peptide): One of the hunger messengers in the brain.

Amino acids: The individual molecules that make up long chains in protein.

Amygdala: Area of the brain involved with the stress response.

Autonomic nervous system: The part of the nervous system that is not under conscious or voluntary control. It is responsible for functions such as blood pressure, heart rate, sweating, etc.

Basal metabolic rate: The rate at which the body expends energy for basic activities of living, including organ function and breathing.

Blood sugar: The concentration of sugar (glucose) molecules in your bloodstream.

Calorie: A measure of the amount of energy available from food.

Carbohydrate: A food type containing chains of sugar molecules.

Cardiovascular: Relating to the heart and blood vessels.

Central nervous system: The main part of the nervous system that includes the spinal cord and brain.

Central obesity: Accumulation of fat around the abdominal or trunk area.

Cholecystokinin (CCK): An important satiety messenger released in the gut when you eat.

Corticotrophin-releasing hormone (CRH): A stress messenger in the brain, which causes an increase in cortisol in the bloodstream.

Cortisol: The body's major stress hormone.

Detoxification: The release and flushing out of harmful toxins from the body.

Dopamine: An important chemical messenger in the brain.

Endocrine glands: Organs of the body containing specialised cells that secrete hormones, e.g. the pancreas, which secretes insulin.

Enkaphalins: A group of chemical messengers involved in the reward system.

Fight-or-flight response: The series of reactions or events designed to help the body handle acute stress.

GABA (gaba-aminobutyric acid): A neurotransmitter involved in the reward system.

Ghrelin: A hunger hormone produced in the stomach, which increases hunger and appetite.

Glucose: Chemical name for the major sugar molecule.

Glycogen: The main storage form of glucose in the liver and muscles.

Hormone: A chemical messenger formed in one part of the body and transported in the blood to a different area where it exerts its effect.

Hunger centre: The region of the brain that when active makes you feel hungry.

Hyperglycaemia: A high concentration of sugar molecules in your bloodstream.

Hyperinsulinaemia: Persistent high insulin levels resulting from a carbohydrate-heavy diet.

Hypoglycaemia: A low concentration of sugar molecules in your bloodstream.

Hypothalamus: Important area of the brain responsible for controlling hunger, satiety and stress.

Inflammation: An aggressive reaction by the body's immune system.

Insulin: Hormone produced by the pancreas that lowers blood sugar and stores fat.

Insulin resistance: A condition in which the body is insensitive and even resistant to the effects of insulin. In most cases the body responds by producing even more insulin, leading to hyperinsulinaemia.

Ketosis: An unhealthy state of starvation for the body.

Leptin: A hormone produced by fat cells that decreases appetite and increases energy expenditure.

Leptin resistance: Resistance of the body to the effects of leptin.

Lipid: Fat or fatty substances including fatty acids, waxes and steroids.

Lipogenesis: The formation of fat, and the transformation of non-fat materials into body fat.

Melatonin: Hormone produced by the pineal gland in the brain.

Metabolic syndrome (syndrome X): A disease complex characterised by central obesity, high blood pressure, insulin resistance, increased cholesterol and increased risk of heart disease and stroke.

Metabolism: Overall term for the ongoing chemical processes in the body that burn food and produce energy.

Naturopathy: Medical practice using natural substances like herbs, foods, acupuncture, etc. to stimulate the body's innate healing response and produce therapeutic effects.

Neuropeptide-Y (NPY): The hunger messenger in the brain that increases hunger, food cravings and fat storage.

Neurotransmitter: A chemical messenger within the brain or nervous system.

Nutritional supplements: Nutritional supplementation is considered the use of vitamins, minerals and herbs for preventive and therapeutic purposes.

Obesity: An excessive accumulation of fat in the body, mainly deposited in the subcutaneous tissues. It is generally considered to occur when a person is 30 per cent or more above normal body weight.

Orexins: A group of appetite-stimulating chemical messengers.

Protein: A food type containing chains of amino acids used for energy and rebuilding the body.

Receptors: Membrane-bound molecules with specific sites for other molecules such as hormones and neurotransmitters to bind into.

Satiety: The sensation of feeling 'full' and no longer hungry.

Satiety centre: The region of the brain that when active makes you feel full.

Serotonin: A chemical messenger important in the control of mood and craving.

Simple carbohydrate: A simple form of sugar such as glucose, lactose and fructose, which is rapidly absorbed into the bloodstream. Includes foods such as bread, potatoes, fruit and sweets.

Index